The Most Noble Diet
Food Selection and Ethics

George Eisman, R.D.

with

Matt Ball, M.S.
Anne Green, Ph.D.

Forward by Michael Klaper, M.D.

Fourth Edition Revised

Publis
Diet
3835
Burdett, NY 14818

D1468634

Copyright 1994

ISBN # 0-9614435-1-0

Library of Congress Catalog Car Number 94-94442

Acknowledgments

I would like to thank Phil Murray for his thorough and insightful editing; Sandra Koski, for her work on previous editions; Irene Cruickshank for her technical assistance; Dr. Michael Klaper for his recommendation of the book to many who have waited for a copy; Harriett Lentz Eisman for her fine editing of this manuscript; and Shelly Schlueter for her illustrations and help in proof-reading. I would also like to thank my son Thomas for being so patient (most of the time) while his dad did this.

Dedicated to all those who live without justice.

Table of Contents

FOREWORD
by Michael Klaper, M.D.

Population explosion ... world hunger ...
threats to personal health ...

These times present a clash of powerful forces that threatens to engulf the individual and the planet itself. We fear losing control of our own lives, and healing the world's momentous problems seems like an impossible dream. We search for solutions, for guideposts, for sanity .... Where to start?

We start with ourselves, of course – we must never forget that each of us has moment-to-moment control over our own thoughts and actions. Indeed, each thought *is* an action. We determine what happens to us and whom we become.

This is especially true when it comes to the food we take into our bodies. What we eat becomes the substance of our material body and determines how well it functions. Food provides both the body's structural building blocks and the fuel upon which the body runs. Both health and disease can be created through our diet; its role in disease creation has become especially evident in my medical practice.

Our American diet, laden with animal fats, produces the illusion of affluence and satisfaction. However, it actually creates the realities of bulging waistlines, clogged arteries, and malignancies of the bowels. During my medical school education, the treatment of diseases was presented with the implication that if the physician could match the right medicine or surgical procedure with the patient's particular disease, the problem would be solved. Mere lip service was given to disease prevention, and almost no recognition was granted to the possible role of diet in the creation of so many of the terrible diseases that occupy so much of the practicing physician's waking hours.

After years spent in the operating room and general practice office, I no longer accept mere medication as the complete treatment of disease. The grim parade of clogged arteries to brain, heart, and legs, the infections of tissues made vulnerable by a weakened immune system, and the malignancies of bowels and skin provoked powerful questions: Why are these things happening to these people? What are they doing that creates such destructive changes in their vital organs? What is out of balance? Is there a common link to all these "different" diseases? Could there be something in "The Great American Diet" that is not actually healthy for Americans?

I spent much of my boyhood on a dairy farm in Wisconsin and was an avid consumer of milk, cheese, ice cream, and other dairy products into my adult years. Under the illusion that milk was "nature's most perfect food," I condoned its use in general diet and recommended it as food for infants. I was quite unaware of the tremendous flux of fat that courses through the blood and body after eating animal products such as meat, eggs, and cheese.

One day when day while drawing blood from a patient, I noticed that the liquid serum part of the blood, normally a beautiful transparent golden yellow, was opaque and creamy white. I asked the man what he had eaten one hour before, and he innocently said, "A cheeseburger and a milk shake," thinking that it was good food. As I visualized his fat-laden blood coursing through his body, profusing every organ and blood vessel large and small, I saw the inevitability of this greasy film layering out on the inside of his arteries, like the "boiler scale" accumulating in a hot water pipe. I saw that this process, repeated several times daily, year after year, was a key mechanism for the terrible collections of fat and cholesterol plaques that clog the arteries of my patients with coronary artery disease, strokes (both "small" and "major"), and ischemic leg pain.

The "riddle" of most cases of high blood pressure then solved itself as I saw how the "piping system" of the body became rigid and narrowed. As in any piping system, narrow arteries increase resistance to flow, thus requiring the heart to pump at higher pressures. This higher pressure then induces further damage to small arteries in the kidney, brain, and heart, as well as wearing out the heart-pump at a faster rate. The subsequent kidney failures, strokes, and heart attacks suddenly became logical and inevitable consequences of a high-fat diet.[1] This was especially likely if other facts predispose, such as genetics, smoking, etc.

As I would treat patients in the office for their high blood pressure and all its concomitant problems, it became obvious that I could not merely prescribe a diuretic or an agent to lower blood pressure without giving guidance as to how to arrest this terrible process from choking off any more vital blood flow. I began to elicit more careful dietary histories from clients, and I became increasingly aware of how each person's diet changes their body. The changes, usually obesity or combined sugar and protein excess, were a main culprit in many "different" diseases. It was easy to see the terrible toll that obesity inflicted upon the body: High blood pressure, heart failure, diabetes, lower back pain, wear-and-tear degeneration of knees and hips, are all caused by or made worse by the encasement of fat. When I asked for a sample of their diet, the origin of the fat became evident: eggs and bacon for breakfast, cheeseburger, fries, and a shake for lunch, steak or hot dogs for dinner with ice cream or baked goods for dessert. The litany was all too familiar, and the appropriateness of "veganizing" their diet was easily seen by most people.

"Stop eating animal fat!" would be repeated throughout my clinical day. More and more, I became a nutritionist and diet planner. To those who were unbelieving that a diet devoid of animal products could leave them with anything to sustain good health, let alone taste good, I could be reassuring.[2] After outlining basic nutritional principles to meet protein and vitamin needs, I joyfully presented highlights of the world of vegan cuisine, from breakfasts of tofu omelets or pancakes, to lunches of hearty soups, sandwiches and salads, through gourmet dinners of lasagnas, Chinese stir-fried vegetables, and "superburgers" (see Appendix E for recipes and other cookbooks). Hearing descriptions of sweet treats like frozen peanut butter "ice cream," carob fudge cookies, and tofu cream

---

[1] "Jack Sprat's Legacy: The Science and Politics of Fats and Cholesterol," Patricia Houseman, Center for Science in the Public Interest, Richard Marek Publishers, New York

[2] *A Vegetarian Sourcebook* , Keith Akers, Vegetarian Press, P.O. Box 61273, Denver, CO 80206.

pie always was reassuring for prospective vegans. Most often, the clients were receptive and enthusiastic. It was as if they already knew the truth of their indulgence in fatty animal foods and were relieved to hear of a logical and delicious solution to their problems and fears.

With the proper substitution of vegan foods, the pounds would just melt away, while the client dined luxuriously on millet burgers and seitan Swiss "steak." The medical charts reflected the beneficial changes; as weights fell, so did blood pressure and the dosages of potent medications needed to control it. Freed from the straight-jacket of obesity, people found they could breathe easier, and walking and other physical activity became a joy again. Both the clients and I celebrated the wonderful changes.

I was able to describe and prescribe the vegan diet with confidence because I had veganized my own diet. I witnesses with joy and amazement how my body became lean and fit, though I ate ample portions at each meal and never really experienced hunger. I understood how, without the continuous influx of saturated animal fats, the body will metabolize much of the fat stored under the skin and adapt to the leaner fuel from plant sources only. Other benefits, such as regular bowel habits, cleaner breath, and lower food budgets, soon became evident. I was eager to share the good news.

However, the vegan diet soon showed itself to benefit many other conditions not overshadowed by obesity. It appears that many states of dis-ease involving low-grade inflammatory reactions (such as rheumatoid arthritis) or skin phenomena such as hives or eczema have an allergic basis that is made worse by many of the proteins introduced by animal foods. Patients with skin disorders and inflamed joints noticed marked relief after discontinuing animal products. Diabetic clients showed the benefits of eating a diet high in whole foods because the complex plant starches and sugars were absorbed into their bloodstream more slowly, allowing for smoother and easier control of their blood sugar. Almost all my clients on insulin or other medicine to lower their blood sugar have been able to reduce their dosages or even eliminate the medicine altogether after they veganized their diet.

One man in my practice had most of his small intestine surgically removed because of repeated attacks of inflammatory bowel disease (Crohn's disease). He was eating the usual American dietary catastrophe and experiencing constant abdominal cramps, diarrhea, and weight loss. While describing a vegan diet to him, I emphasized the use of tofu because it is an excellent protein source and very easily digestible. The results were rapid and dramatic – the pain and diarrhea ceased, he gained weight, and he once again felt like a healthy man.

The anecdotes go on and on, all attesting to something profoundly right about the human body running on a fuel free of the blood and flesh of animals.

At the same time, I began encountering analyses in the media of the problem of world hunger. The numbers that explain the present grim situation of mass starvation in half the globe are clear, and actually point the way to a world of plenty.

As anyone who has ever studied ecology knows, converting plant protein and energy to animal flesh is inefficient and wasteful. The acreage required to feed one person a pound of meat daily for one year, if the land is instead planted with high-protein staple crops such as soybeans, grains, and garden vegetables, could nourish fifteen people. More than ample farmland is available on the planet if it is used to grow food for people, not beef cattle. However, about 85% of the corn, 80% of the soybeans, and 90% oats grown in the United States are fed to livestock destined to become slaughtermeat! In this sense, the Most Noble Diet – the vegan diet – becomes even more noble.

In addition, a vegan diet would also eliminate one of the darkest blights against humanity's belief in our own nobility – the massive cruelty that is inflicted upon the innocent animals whose blood and flesh we consume daily. Every day in the United States, over nineteen million animals will be killed, the vast majority for food.

Besides the concentrated poisoning of their flesh with pesticides and other toxins from feed grains, as well as hormones to increase bulk production, the animals are kept in cruel conditions on factory farms where the only thought is on the production of profit. Even the dairy and egg industries have the animals' blood on their hands because all the stock animals are sent for slaughter as soon as their milk or egg production

The Most Noble Diet

falls off. If everyone on the planet consumed the Most Noble Diet, this unspeakable cruelty and exploitation would fade from the planet. Those who presently earn their livelihood from slaughter-related food production, some of the harshest jobs in this country, could be helped to convert to production of other staple food products, such as growing soybeans or producing tofu or texturized vegetable protein.

In addition, the vegan diet would promote the elimination of the economic imbalance that stems from the Western taste for animal flesh and imported delicacies. This would lead to more just food distribution, ease international tensions between the "have" and the "have not" nations, and lead the way toward world peace.

In the following pages, Mr. George Eisman, R.D., provides an excellent analysis of the different aspects of how diet affects and determines the fate of the individual, and at this time in history, the fate of the planet itself. Saving the world may not be your primary concern, but saving yourself should be. I have seen how the vegan diet is a lifesaver, and could be a world-saver. I urge you to discover what you can do to gain health and happiness (not to mention delicious eating) through the Most Noble Diet.

Note: Dr. Klaper is a graduate of the University of Illinois Medical School, and is now a practicing physician in the State of Florida. He is the author of two books: *Vegan Nutrition: Pure and Simple,* and *Pregnancy, Children, and the Vegan Diet.*

INTRODUCTION

Food is a necessity of life; it is one of the cruelest of circumstances when a person starves to death. Even the most sinister of criminals is fed adequate meals while in prison, right up until the bountiful "last meal" before execution, which must be seen as an unimaginable waste by the millions of people, mostly children, who die each year around the world because they cannot get enough to eat.

If any of these hungry people were your neighbors, unemployed and trying to grow their own food, you would certainly share generously what you have to at least guarantee their survival. No moral person would consider stealing food from their neighbor's meager backyard garden. Yet, on a global scale, this thievery happens daily.

Although we ostensibly "buy" agricultural items grown in the poorer countries of the world, those most impoverished obviously do not benefit, for their cycle of poverty continues. The citizens of the country become poorer while the rich nations outbid them for their own produce.

The environmental slogan "Think Globally, Act Locally" could also be written as "Think Globally by Buying Locally." In the United States, we can easily feed ourselves with produce grown in our own country. This not only allows other countries to better feed their own citizens, but supports our local farm population, which has withered from the pressures of industrialization and consolidation. In other countries, buying locally is also preferable. If some agricultural items must be imported, these products should come only from countries that are able to feed their own citizens adequately.

This book is not political – I take only the side of feeding all people. This is and has been my oath of service as a professional nutritionist and dietitian. Labels such as capitalist, communist, left, right, white, black, Christian, Jew, Muslim, atheist have no meaning when it comes to starving children or

The Most Noble Diet

malnourished pregnant women. There is just food, and the land to grow that food.

If we can all just realize this simple fact for one moment, and stop fighting over the land that holds the roots that support the tree that bears the fruit that feeds the child, then maybe, just maybe ... peace.

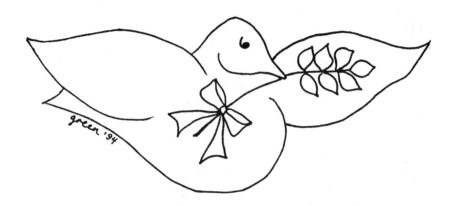

CHAPTER 1
FOOD CHOICES

We all have to eat. What we choose to eat depends on a variety of factors, which are generally divided into two concerns: availability and acceptability. In the United States today, availability is mainly a function of affordability – if you can afford it, you can get any food, anywhere, anytime, with few exceptions. In making good choices, we can decide where to shop or dine, what to buy or order, based on what we want and what we can afford. Seasonality of certain produce items influences availability for most of us (we learn not to expect fresh watermelon in January), but far more influential is the price of food relative to money available.

Some say that the world's hunger problem is not one of food shortage, but rather a problem of poverty. In reality, these are the same thing, since the foods are not available at the price the hungry people can afford. This concept will be addressed further in following chapters; for now, we will dismiss the availability issue as mainly a matter of money.

Next is the concept of acceptability, which can in turn be broken into a social component and an individual component. In a social, or group, context the acceptability of certain foods can be a religious matter and/or a cultural convention. For example, devout Moslems and Jews everywhere do not eat pork for religious reasons; for cultural conformity, Americans and Europeans do not eat dogs or cats. Except for a few tribal societies, there is a universal disdain for cannibalism, usually through a combination of religious, cultural, and legal taboos.

The acceptability of a new food, such as an exotic fruit or an unusual (food-wise) breed of animal is, to a large extent, determined by its similarity to familiar items. In cosmopolitan societies like the United States, individual choice (heavily assaulted by advertising) is the ultimate determinant of incorporation into the set of acceptable "eats." The social

The Most Noble Diet

aspects of food acceptability, then, usually deal with labeling certain items as undesirable, and from among the remaining potential foods, our personal concept of individual acceptability dictates which (and how much) of these foods will constitute our actual diet.

In making our individual food choices from that set of foods already determined to be financially available and socially acceptable, there is a hierarchy of motivational principles that can guide us. Other than those being tube-fed in a comatose state, conscious and free-living adults use this hierarchy to guide their food choices.

Since you are reading this page, I will assume that you are at least somewhat conscious. The "consciousness" concept is very much (over)worked by a segment of the population in discussing individual "enlightenment" or self-fulfillment. In the present context, there are similar overtones, but the desired implication is that in a more mundane spirit of caring and responsibility, we are the masters of our own destinies and, in a collective sense, the destiny of the planet.

The six levels of progressively conscious concerns that underlie individual acceptability in diet selection are

- Hedonism: eating what you enjoy for sensual gratification
- Personal Health: eating what you believe is "good" for you
- Environment: eating what the Earth provides without undue disturbance to ecosystems
- Politics: eating (or not eating) as a statement against specific oppressive actions or policies
- Nonviolence: eating only what can be obtained without intentional injury or cruelty
- Humanity: eating only what is your "fair share" in this global human community; that is, not demanding extravagances that deprive other individuals of their basic requirements of life

The remainder of this book discusses each of these concerns as they are experienced today. The purpose of eating is to provide sustenance for your body. I have no intention of instilling guilt over every mouthful of food that is taken from a lower level of consciousness motivation. In my professional practice as a nutrition consultant, I have encountered many people paralyzed with fear over eating almost any food, lest it do harm to them or another. This book is an attempt to help you choose the best diet for yourself, your community, and your planet, in the context of your continued energetic survival. The lesson is not all the things you "cannot" do, but rather that you can take action to make the world a better place.

If you have any concern that you are compromising your health or the health of any of your family members, I strongly suggest that you consult a recognized nutrition professional, identifiable by licensed status from an official sanctioning agency. In the United States, the American Dietetic Association is that agency, and the status of Registered Dietitian (R.D.) is granted those who have systematically studied the science of nutrition as it relates to disease therapy.

Many self-proclaimed "nutritionists" offer prolific advice, but with few exceptions are unable to differentiate scientifically proven fact from theoretical conjecture. The R.D., or equivalent in other countries, is not only trained to separate fact from fantasy, but is morally obligated by professional ethics to respect the client's food-related belief system.[3] To contact a Registered Dietitian in your area, call your hospital's Dietary Department and ask for the number of the Dietetic Association for your locality.

---

[3] *The Journal of the American Dietetic Association*, 1980, vol. 77, p. 68.

The Most Noble Diet

CHAPTER 2
HEDONISM: FOOD AND PLEASURE

The belief that the chief good of humanity lies in the pursuit of pleasure was the guiding principle of the Hedonist school of ancient Greek philosophers. This philosophy can be seen in the children of all societies, who develop a preference for individual foods based on looks, smell, texture, taste, even sound. "Snap-Crackle-Pop" can be a welcome noise for children when no one else will talk to them (serves them right for wanting breakfast at 6 a.m. on a Saturday).

Choosing foods on the basis of their appeal to our five senses continues into adulthood, but this philosophy is generally frowned upon as immature and irresponsible as the sole basis for diet selection. As we "grow up," we are supposed to concentrate our diet selections on what is good for us; this will be addressed in Chapter 3.

It is not my intention to condemn the hedonistic approach to food selection; after all, it is a basic instinct of the human animal. What will emerge, however, is that at this point in time, conditions exist that have the potential to have negative consequences if one follows the hedonistic instincts without temperance and reason.

The Five Senses

To some extent, each of the five senses is used in selecting items that might be appealing as a meal or a snack. Other animals, of course, use their senses as well, but to differing degrees than we do. A dog, for example, will sniff everything potentially edible (which, for some dogs, is everything). We, of course, use our vision to disqualify many items before letting them get that close to our noses.

Taste. Our tongues have only four different types of taste buds. We distinguish sweet, salty, bitter, and sour flavors within our mouths.[4] Other "flavors" are determined by a combination of these four flavors and our sense of smell.

Overall, the sense of taste does not play as great a role in the food selection process as one might think, because by the time the food has gotten to the mouth it has usually passed the acceptability test of at least one of the other four senses. The tongue acts more as a last line of defense against the failure of our other senses.

The best example of this is the sensation of sweetness, which is determined by the taste buds on the front tip of the tongue. The placement of these sweetness receptors suggests that they act as indicators of whether or not to eat the item. In nature, ripe fruits are much sweeter than unripe ones, and not nearly so sickly sweet as the rotten fruits. Even fully-ripened fruits[5] begin to lose their sweetness as they are stored for any period of time. Try an ear of freshly-picked corn sometime, raw, right off the cob (wash it first), but save a bit for later. The change over time is unmistakable, as the sugars are turned into starch. Heat can turn starches back into sugars to some extent, which is why we usually cook our corn (at the expense of some nutrients).

In the grocery store, however, thousands of products exist with sweeteners added to compensate for the lack of freshness. This use of sweeteners to simulate the flavor of freshness of course has a negative side, starting with tooth decay. Just as heating or other processing causes the loss of some nutrients in foods, adding sugar to them creates the same result. Refined sugars are "empty calories" in that there is substance to be digested and metabolized, but without the accompanying nutrients that facilitate the digestive processes. Refined sugar can thus rob the body of vitamins, especially B-vitamins, by forcing the use of accumulated stores. This can set the stage for overt diseases of deficiency (which are not very common), sub-clinical conditions (which are probably very common),

---

[4] Some Oriental systems proclaim a fifth mouth-distinguished flavor they call pungent. It is similar to what we call spicy hot, which does seem to be determined in the mouth. One cannot smell the "heat" of peppers, it just sneaks up on you. However, many people in Western cultures would be hard-pressed to call this experience a flavor.

[5] I use the term fruits loosely, in the sense of "fruit of the earth," to indicate any edible part of the plant.

The Most Noble Diet

and certainly a lack of reserves for times of true emergencies. Fooling Mother Nature – our taste – has its costs.

Smell. While choosing and eating something, we smell it. The old adage "You taste what you smell" can be demonstrated by sniffing an onion while biting into an apple. What we miss during a cold reminds us of how often we use our sense of smell.[6]

For some, the aromas of brewing coffee, baking cookies (especially chocolate chip), and sizzling bacon are strong temptations to consume. But these smells exist only because of significant alterations of the substances involved.[7] Fragrances in nature are generally subtle; it is the flowers, not always the edible portions, that are the most powerfully fragrant. It is usually not until we break into the fruit with our hands or teeth that the smell is released.

The smell of something is determined by substances called essential oils, which are fat-soluble substances. These can be released by simple heating, but even more so by frying in some type of fat. That is why french fries smell so much better than boiled potatoes, but at quite a cost in terms of empty calories (in this case fat calories) added.

When we get a cold, we are often told to avoid "mucus-producing" foods such as milk-fat. The fact that we can no longer smell (and be tempted by) fatty foods might lead us to eat more subtly-flavored foods like fresh fruits and vegetables. It is interesting to note that fresh fruits and vegetables used to be referred to as "protective foods" because of their high vitamin and mineral content. *Sometimes* our sensual instincts are our guides to health.

Touch and Hearing. These two senses are addressed together because in regard to food we often use our sense of

---

[6] Perhaps by letting us get sick, nature is telling us not to eat so much of something that might have placed our system out of balance.

[7] Few people find the smell of a pig on a farm or in a slaughterhouse appetizing. It is in our reaction to non-processed animal flesh that human beings' true herbivorous nature is best seen. The digestive juices of human beings do not begin to flow at the sight of a cow or pig. And the sight of an animal being killed is actually repulsive and even nauseating to most people, rather than appetizing. But who is repulsed by seeing an apple picked from a tree or a carrot taken from the ground?

hearing as a guide to the texture of things we haven't yet touched. This is frequently demonstrated on television and radio commercials when we hear the magnified "crunch" of potato or corn chips, allegedly as proof of their crisp texture. In nature, a crisp texture is a sign of freshness (think of an apple or carrot). With chemical manipulation, however, some processed foods can be made to stay crisp for months, even years. Few would want to eat a four-month-old baked potato, yet that is considered the "shelf life" of potato chips.

The sense of touch is used in food selection in two ways: mouth-feel and hand-feel. We use our hands to squeeze melons, tomatoes, peaches, and loaves of bread to discern softness. Freshness, however, can be manipulated by commercial processors. For example, a loaf of bread is usually soft when fresh, and it hardens as it becomes stale. Many chemicals are added to commercial bread to keep them soft long after their freshness is gone. The traditional bakeries sold day-old bread at a discount, while today supermarkets are filled with day(s) old bread at full price.

On the other hand, a fruit starts out too hard, softens, and eventually becomes too soft (rotten). Wax coatings and other treatments are applied to most of the produce sold in regular food markets. This is done to keep the vegetables and fruits firm as long as possible. One of the reasons store-bought tomatoes don't taste like home grown is that they are picked when extremely green, artificially ripened with gases, and then kept at cold temperatures to prevent spoilage. This process retards the flavor development that occurs in the natural ripening process, and allows them to get old without being obviously rotten.

Sight. It is our sense of sight that human beings depend most heavily for decision-making, including food selection. It is significant that blind people generally develop a more acute sense of hearing, but deaf people do not develop more acute vision (in fact, they often get eye strain from having to read lips). This is because we already use our sense of sight so fully.

Both color and form are important qualities used to discern what looks good to eat. It is not just on a whim that children's drinks are brightly colored (artificially, in most cases); children tend to prefer them this way, often believing that they taste better. Artificial coloring is added to many other products as well, such as the skin of fruits, on the premise that adults prefer brightly colored foods as well. However, in nature fruits can be ripe before they lose all the green from their skins; in fact, they are often overripe when completely colored.

The form of foods is also significant to their appeal. We tend to prefer shapes that are roughly symmetrical and have a firm, solid appearance (such as a cantaloupe). Most people are tempted by the sight of a perfect hot fudge sundae. But let the ice cream melt for just a few moments, and it will be a gooey, runny mess that calls for a mop instead of a spoon. The taste would still be about the same, but the change in appearance and texture has altered its appeal.

In conclusion, our senses crave fresh food. To fool the senses by eating foods that are artificially manipulated to resemble freshness is to enjoy false pleasures. The price for this deception is exacted in the future, be it a headache twenty minutes later or the development of cancer twenty years later. Fresh foods that are instinctively appealing to us turn out to be hedonistically, as well as logically, the best choice of foods.

CHAPTER 3
HEALTH

Moving beyond personal pleasure, we go from foods we like to foods that are good for us. Herein lies the conflict that haunts many people these days, because there is so much controversy over what is truly the most healthful diet. In addition, there is also a pervasive sentiment that things that taste good are probably not good for you. This is the choice we are given as adults: to be responsible and concerned with our personal well-being or to live recklessly. It generally makes life a little easier for those close to us if we remain healthy, but for the most part, it is only we as individuals who will benefit or suffer health effects from our food choices.

It is not necessary to be extremely self-health conscious in order to go on to higher levels of noble thinking and action, but some measure of bodily self-respect is needed to preserve total well-being. For example, there are many "junk food" vegetarians who abstain from eating animal flesh for humanitarian reasons (see following chapters) rather than for hygienic concerns. Yet if these people suffer ill health, they are not only handicapped in the efforts to create a gentler, more just world, but they also set a poor example for those who may be considering changing their diet in a similar direction. This is especially true when those influenced are concerned parents.

Getting the Goods from Foods

All food comes from life (except for some rock derivatives, like salt, which really isn't a food because it provides no energy). Fresh food is the closest to its life-source. The further food is removed from its source, the more nutrition tends to be removed or lost as the food's constituents break down in a process commonly called rotting.

In nature, rotting is an essential process that renews the soil for the next generation of plants. However, except for the grubworms among us, we prefer to consume foods before the rotting process goes too far. With modern technology, there are methods to slow down this process, but, as noted in the previous chapter, there is always a price to pay for fooling our instincts.

All vitamins and all energy nutrients – the ones that contain calories (carbohydrates, fats, and proteins) – are organic[8] molecules. Chemically speaking, this means that they all contain carbon atoms in a certain configuration. Practically speaking, it means they are subject to breakdown and loss of their nutritive benefit. This breakdown is caused by factors such as exposure to air, light, heat, and chemical/biological processes involving acids, bases, or enzymes.

The minerals in foods (such as iron, calcium, and zinc) are inorganic molecules; just as the medieval alchemists could not change iron into gold, these nutrients do not break down into other things. However, there is the possibility of the minerals being leached out into water (which is why if you cook vegetables in water, the liquid ought to be saved for a soup base). In addition, the minerals may be rendered unavailable to the body because they are bound to certain chemicals. Thus, processing foods will lose or change some of the things we need from the foods.

Trying to replenish what is lost is a distant second to the best option of just eating the intact original product. There are two approaches to replenishment of lost nutrition in the preserving and processing of foods, and both have their shortcomings.

Ré-enriching. The first approach, done largely because of government regulation, is to re-enrich the food with major nutrients, the lack of which has caused health problems for people in the past. Thus, iron, thiamin, riboflavin, and niacin are added to grain products such as flour. They are then marketed as "enriched" products. There are, however, many more nutrients lost in the refining process that are not added back, and the health consequences of these lacks in the Western diet are becoming apparent.

---

[8] This is a different use of the word organic than will be referred to later in a discussion of "organically-grown" produce.

When foods are processed, two things happen, both of which are good for the industry's profits. One is that value is added to the product (from a purely economic standpoint, certainly not from a nutritional standpoint). This means that more can be charged for the product, creating more profit.

Second, the more nutritious a product is, the more attractive it is to other organisms, and thus more prone to spoilage. Refining changes the product to make it less nutritious, meaning that there will be less spoilage, greater shelf-life, and thus greater profit. To suggest that all nutrients that are refined away be added back is to suggest that processing ought not to have been done in the first place. The food-processing industry lobby knows that unprocessed food, on the whole, is the best choice nutritionally, but they also know that if this word got out, they would be out of business. Thus, they will fight to make certain that enrichment regulations lag far behind nutritional science.

Vitamin B-6 (pyridoxine) is an excellent case in point. This nutrient, essential for red blood cell formation as well as a host of other important bodily processes, is lost in the milling of white flour.[9] A slice of whole wheat bread contains about three times as much B-6 as a slice of white bread. None is added back in the "enriching" process (which would be better termed the "partially re-enriching" process). A vitamin B-6 deficiency in adult human beings can cause nervousness, irritability, weakness, and insomnia.[10] There are serious flaws in thinking that enrichment is an adequate solution to food adulteration, and the enrichment process will always remain a "finger in the dam" solution, with the added complication that it takes years of struggle for regulations to mandate that another finger be used when a new leak is spotted.

Pill Popping. The other approach to making a good diet out of impoverished food is by taking vitamin and mineral pills. It is true that vitamin and mineral preparations sold without a prescription are not hazardous when taken as directed on the

---

[9] To be perfectly fair, B-6 was not discovered until about seven years after the enrichment program was mandated. However, over fifty years later, there is still no required vitamin B-6 enrichment of refined grains; regulations are slow, if not impossible, to change.

[10] As can many conditions. Please do not self-diagnose.

label, but many so-called "health" magazines recommend dosages far in excess of the label instructions. This is because the labels are regulated to an extent by the Food and Drug Administration, which prohibits recommending harmful dosages, but the magazines are protected by the First Amendment, allowing them to publish anyone's opinion. The consequences of these opinions are carried out to an almost comedic extreme by individuals who pull out a shoe-box full of bottles each morning for their daily swallowing ritual – spray enough bullets into the air and you are bound to hit at least one mosquito. In other words, these people think that any possible deficiency will surely be helped if you take everything. I have termed this outlook the "nuclear bomb" approach to nutrition: the bomb may well wipe out the enemy, but the side effects may be worse than coexisting with the initial problem!

One problem with this approach is that we do not yet know what "everything" is. New nutrients are continuously being discovered, and others are being refuted. Vitamin peddlers will always push the "total" panacea for the 90s, which is different than it was in the 80s, which is different from the 70s, etc. The fervor to keep up to date is unquestionable. But in the frenzy to lengthen the vitamin and mineral shopping list, the interrelationships among the nutrients are being ignored.

The fact that our bodies use nutrients in conjunction with each other has long been apparent.[11] It is indeed a questionable practice to take huge doses of anything, except in response to a specific disorder. A multi-vitamin pill or a box full of different pills are undoubtedly missing things that have not yet been discovered; by taking large amounts of everything else, you may be increasing your body's need for these unknown factors. But if you do not take these pills, your body can receive the unknowns in sufficient amounts and combinations from fresh, whole foods. It is possible that new nutrients will be discovered by observations of deficiency symptoms in pill-overdosers; if you care more about advancing knowledge in the

---

[11] For some of the complex interrelationships that have been observed, the serious student is referred to *Micronutrient Interactions: Vitamins, Minerals, and Hazardous Element*, edited by O. A. Levander and Lorraine Cheng, New York, N.Y. Academy of Sciences, 1980.

science of nutrition than you care about your own health, keep popping 'em.

Poisons in Your Food?

Beyond losing the good from food, many bads often appear in foods, such as pesticides, herbicides, preservatives, additives, mineral-binders, cholesterol, and saturated fats.[12] Reading labels never tells the entire story, for not all possible contaminants are listed, or even tested.

Plant Foods. Pesticide and herbicide residuals are not just a worry for fresh produce, but can be found in many foods that come from farms that follow the chemical approach to growing food. Although it is important that we all lobby the government for stricter monitoring of farming and food-processing practices, the immediate solution is to deal directly with the growers. When purchasing direct, one can seek out unsprayed products when possible, even offering to pay more (which is cheaper than hospital bills).

Preservatives are added to foods to keep them edible longer. The chemicals used are poisonous in large quantities, but their effects on human beings when ingested in smaller amounts over a long period of time are basically unknown. The most common preservatives used in bread and other baked goods are propionates (calcium and sodium propionate). It is interesting (though not conclusive) that the symptoms of a Vitamin B-12 deficiency become apparent when propionate acid accumulates in the body, causing long nerve cell damage. Vitamin B-12 is that vitamin that is technically not found in a strict vegetarian diet, yet several reports exist showing many strict vegetarians from India and Pakistan who had no signs of this deficiency until they moved to a more "civilized" country – one that puts preservatives in commercial breads. Alternatives to chemical preservatives are storage in air-tight containers, or freezing. Of course, the best alternative is actual freshness.

Additives to food include colorings, flavorings, dough conditioners, drying agents, moisturizers, and thickeners. They are generally listed on labels, but beware that a food can be

---

[12] In addition to human and animal genes inserted into the genetic code for produce, and hormones in animal foods.

The Most Noble Diet

labeled NO PRESERVATIVES, and yet in small letters around the side list a number of chemical ingredients added for other purposes. All of these additives are just used to help simulate the look, smell, texture, and taste of a fresher product. Again, the safest way is the freshest way.

Much has been written about mineral-binders that naturally occur in foods like whole wheat and spinach. These binders, namely oxalates and phytates, inhibit the absorption of some of the minerals in foods. This is the type of information food manufacturers like to use when defending the use of additives. "What's wrong with putting additives in foods when these detrimental substances are naturally there?" they argue. It is also fuel for the health-food store pill-pushers to claim superiority for their "purified" mineral preparations. The truth is that only a small amount of the minerals in question are unavailable. By no means is the food rendered worthless, and it is certainly not harmful to include these foods in one's diet.

Animal Products. Contamination is a much greater problem with animal products than with plant foods for a number of reasons. Pesticides, herbicides, and other toxins in the environment concentrate in animal fat, building up as one eats higher on the food chain. Even if there are potentially harmful pesticides on our plant crops (which can be washed), it still makes more sense to eat the grain itself than to eat the flesh of cows who have spent years ingesting hundreds of pounds of grain sprayed and unwashed, all the while incorporating toxic residues into their fat and vital organs.[13] Even so-called "organic" meat may come from animals that are not fed organically-grown grains. Obviously, these animal products cannot be rinsed off in hopes of making them safer.

In addition to these contaminants in the animals' feed, the animals are given a number of drugs to keep them alive in intensive confinement. A Congressional study found that as many as 90% or more of the tens of thousands of new animal drugs estimated to be on the market have not been approved by the FDA. In addition, as many as 4,000 of these drugs have "potentially significant adverse effects on animals or

---

[13] An in-depth review of the health hazards of foods from animal sources can be found in *The Animal Connection* by Agatha Thrash, M.D., and Calvin Thrash, M.D. (Seale, AL.: Yuchi Pines Institute, 1983)

humans."[14] Over half of all antibiotics used each year in the United States are fed to animals destined to be slaughtered and consumed. This practice was banned in the 1970s by the European Economic Community, because it leads to more resistant strains of bacteria. Despite all the drugs, these animals are not healthy. According to the *Atlanta Constitution*, "Every week throughout the South, millions of chickens leaking yellow pus, stained by green feces, contaminated by harmful bacteria, or marred by lung and heart infection, cancerous tumors or skin conditions are shipped to consumers."[15] Bacterial contamination of animal products regularly kills many people throughout the United States every year.

Cholesterol is a type of fat that is found significantly only in animal flesh (including fish), dairy products, and eggs, as well as in clogged arteries of people who have heart attacks and strokes. Because of this, cholesterol has become a food "villain." Eating a lot of cholesterol-containing foods is one unhealthy practice in this regard, but there is another, even more significant factor: eating saturated fat. Saturated fat is the common fat in animal products and in a few vegetable oils. Generally those fats that are solid at room temperature are composed mostly of saturated fat.

The miracle of modern technology has enabled food manufacturers to turn unsaturated fats into saturated fats by a process called hydrogenation. The result – a hydrogenated or hardened fat – can be just as detrimental as any saturated fat, but leaves us subject to being fooled by labels that tout such claims as "100% Corn Oil" margarine. Corn oil is mostly unsaturated, but it is hydrogenated in the process of making margarine. Such hydrogenated fats are added to most commercial peanut butters in order to keep them from separating. The manufacturers then have the nerve to label the jar NO CHOLESTEROL even though the hardened fats added have an even worse effect on the body, causing it to increase cholesterol production. The only peanut butter that does not have added hydrogenated fat is the "natural kind." These separate in the jar and should be refrigerated after opening.

---

[14] *Human Food Safety and Animal Drugs*, 1985.
[15] May 26, 1991.

The Most Noble Diet

Diseases of the West

While nutritional science has traditionally focused on avoiding deficiencies, the truth is that most diseases in western societies are diseases of excess, rather than of deficiency. According to the American Dietetic Association, people who do not eat animal flesh have a lower risk of heart disease, stroke, colon cancer, osteoporosis, diabetes milletus, obesity, kidney stones, gallstones, hypertension, and possibly breast cancer.[16] A brief summary of some of these diseases follows.

Heart Disease is the number one killer in the United States. It has been shown that heart disease is correlated with elevated levels of cholesterol, which is found only in animal products. T. Colin Campbell of Cornell University showed that Chinese men, who consume an average of less than 2 ounces of meat per day, have an average cholesterol level of 127 mg/dl, and their risk of heart disease is 1/16 that of a typical American male. As with other diseases, when the Chinese adopt a Western diet, they are subject to the same levels of heart disease.

Colon Cancer is the number two cause of cancer deaths in the United States. Meat eating and a lack of dietary fiber are linked to colon cancer. Animal products contain no fiber – only plants do.

Osteoporosis (loss of bone calcium) has been shown to be linked to excessive protein intake, which is common in people who eat an animal-based diet. Campbell's study, mentioned above, showed that Americans have twice the incidence of osteoporosis that the Chinese have, despite the fact that we consume twice the calcium, 3/4 of which comes from dairy products. Most Chinese get their calcium from green leafy vegetables and whole-grain cereal crops; almost none drink the milk of animals.

Avoiding Overeating

What is most ignored about foods is what it is that makes us stop eating various things even though we may not be "full." Have you noticed during fruit seasons you can eat oranges or

---

[16] ADA Position Paper on Vegetarian Diets.

apples until you just couldn't take another bite, yet other times have eaten a typical big meal and still had room for dessert? Chances are you'd eaten only a couple hundred calories of fruit, but the big meal might have contained five times that amount. Fresh fruits and vegetables are mostly water, and they contain fiber, both of which fill us up. There seem to be other factors as well that provide an automatic turn-off when we eat too much of any one fruit or vegetable. This is a great feature for those of us who don't want to overeat. The tragic thing is that these factors are either removed or altered during the processing of food, thereby allowing us to overeat the finished products. For those who are underweight, eating a variety of fresh foods will circumvent these natural turn-offs. For overweight people, making a meal of just one kind of fresh fruit or vegetable, such as oranges or carrots, provides a simple way to restrict calories.

Balancing the Diet

The human body needs a source of energy to maintain itself We measure this energy in units called calories. We can get calories from four different categories of nutrients: fats, proteins, carbohydrates, and alcohol. The other categories of nutrients – vitamins, minerals, and water – are all vital but provide no energy. Alcohol in excess causes destruction of brain cells as well as liver tissue, so it should be dismissed as a good source of energy. The other three categories – fats, proteins, and carbohydrates – are thus what we must rely on for fuel.

The body needs a small amount of fat (known as essential fatty acids) and a moderate, but still relatively small amount of protein (essential amino acids) for building body tissues. All of these can easily be gotten from foods of plant origin (grains, vegetables, fruits). All additional fats and proteins eaten, beyond the required amount, are dismantled and burned for energy (calories) but with a price to pay. This excess of fat and protein as energy sources is the primary imbalance in the Western diet.

Most people in the United States have been brainwashed by our food industries and their cohorts in the USDA to believe that the "Four Food Groups" were somehow bequeathed to us by nature as the right way to eat. As 9 of the 10 leading causes of death in the United States are related to dietary imbalances, it seems time to rethink this position. The Food Pyramid, finally unveiled to the pubic in 1993, is an improvement in the proper direction, but still gives the idea that animal products are necessary in the diet.

The Four Food Groups were developed after World War II to help deal with the excess dairy production in the United States. Thus, cows' milk and its derivatives were given exclusive status as a group unto itself, of which everyone was supposed to partake several times daily. That's a good strategy to sell something. However, the "necessity" of milk was not always promoted so strongly. For example, less than twenty years earlier, because children need more Vitamin D than adults it had been mandated that milk be the source for Vitamin D fortification because children drank it and adults did not. Adults who consume excess milk may risk bone loss from this excessive (for them) fortification.

The inappropriateness of recommending that everyone drink milk is not the only thing wrong with the Four Food Groups as a diet-balancing method. The most serious flaw is its over-emphasis on foods that contain too much fat, too much protein, or both. Most people now realize that too much fat, especially animal fat, is unhealthy and is related to heart disease, strokes, and certain common cancers. What most people still don't realize, however, is that excess protein, especially animal protein,[17] is also unhealthy; it is related to kidney failure, liver disease, osteoporosis, some cancers, and even heart disease.

The Four Food Groups, and now the Pyramid, promote two entire groups of foods (dairy and meat) that by nature provide mainly fat and protein. By selecting "lean" meats and "low-fat" dairy products from these groups, consumers are doing nothing more than increasing their relative protein intake, thus trading one set of diseases for another. Because chicken flesh is lower in calories than "red" meats, it contains four times more cholesterol per calorie than beef or pork.

The only energy nutrient that is not toxic in excess is carbohydrates (sugars and starches with their associated

---

[17] In fact, independent of fat and cholesterol intake, many studies have recently shown the link between animal protein and heart disease. See "Healthy Hearts: The Whole Story," V. Messina, M.P.H., R.D., *Good Medicine*, Winter, 1994.

fiber), and this nutrient was found only in the other two "groups": Breads & Cereals and Fruits & Vegetables. The best feature of the Food Pyramid is that these foods are heavily endorsed by being the bases of the pyramid (although some believe that this positioning accords breads, cereals, fruits, and vegetables a psychologically "lower" status).[18]

Most breads are made from cereal grains. The old saying that "Bread is the staff of life" was no faddist health claim. Every civilization before our modern Western society had a diet based on grain products and suffered none of the diseases caused by energy nutrient imbalance. Most of our diet should come from foods made up of complex carbohydrates. Many truly fad "diets" in recent decades ignored carbohydrates, sometimes with tragic results. Diets that stress protein and/or fat for weight loss (or anything else) are simply ignoring human physiology and flirting with serious illness or death. Some diets are intended to induce sickness as a means of suppressing appetite – not a good trade-off.

A diet rich in complex carbohydrates, including fiber (in other words, a plant-based diet) is health supporting and weight controlling.[19] Plants are certainly more desirable sources of nourishment than are animals. Foods from animals (meat, fish, eggs, dairy products) have no fiber and tend to be high in fat and protein, overdoses of which have been found to be associated with hardening of the arteries and/or cancer. The American Cancer Society's February 1984 Report, for instance, recommends the following changes in the typical American diet to help prevent cancer:

• Eating less fat from meat and dairy products, as well as less salt-cured, smoked, and charcoal-broiled meat.

• Eating more: raw vegetables, whole grains, fruits, green vegetables, and cabbage family vegetables (broccoli, cauliflower, cabbage, turnips).

As will be expounded in the following chapters, choosing plants as a food source over animals has the added advantages of being less wasteful of natural resources, less cruel to our

---

[18] In the Pyramid, fruits and vegetables are divided into separate groups in the hope of encouraging more consumption. However, the distinction between the two is merely culinary.

[19] See *Eat More, Weigh Less*, Dean Ornish, M.D.

The Most Noble Diet

fellow creatures, and more compassionate to the people who produce our food.

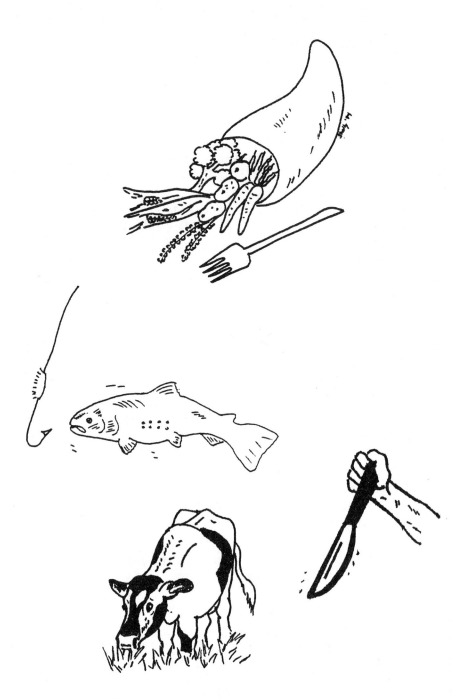

CHAPTER 4
THE ENVIRONMENT

The first widespread public outcry in the United States against the destruction of the natural environment from the use of agricultural chemicals was in the early 1960s and was largely a result of Rachel Carson's in depth exposé *Silent Spring*.[20] Pesticides such as DDT have subsequently been banned for use in this country,[21] based on the idea that growing more food cheaply is not worth the trade-off of losing entire species of wildlife.

Individuals who choose not to eat foods grown with pollutive substances are expressing a concern not only for their health, but for their habitat. Although there is an unresolved controversy as to whether "organically grown" foods (those produced without any synthetic chemicals) have a greater nutritive value than those grown with synthetic fertilizers, pesticides, and/or herbicides, avoiding substances that linger lethally in soil, water, and air is certainly less disruptive to the environmental balance. By operating on this higher level of "nobility," we can choose to take the less damaging option with respect to the world in which we live.

Because there is no evidence indicating that organically grown foods are at all lacking relative to other foods, the only issues are cost and convenience. As demand for these foods increases, they become less costly and more readily accessible, as can be discovered in any university town where co-op stores serve a student community with a large environmental movement.

Another side of this issue is the waste disposal problem. In this country, we are literally drowning in our own garbage. Much of what we dump in huge piles, bury at sea, or burn into

---

[20] Fawcett World Library, 1962

[21] Many chemicals that are illegal in the United States are allowed to be exported for use in other countries, where they can be used on foods which are then exported.

the atmosphere is usable organic matter – like yard trimmings and kitchen wastes of plant origin. Instead of polluting with them, we ought to put a premium on their re-use in our growing fields by supporting organic methods of fertilization by our farmers. Working relationships between city-dwellers and farmers, in which natural refuse is used as fertilizer, can be pursued on a small or large scale. City folk would reduce their solid waste disposal problem, and farmers would reduce their fertilizer cost, but it would be our environment that would be the greatest benefactor.

A third issue of environmental concern in regard to food production is the unnecessary burning of fossil fuels (gasoline, diesel, etc.) used to transport foods over long distances. It is not just the use of the fuel that is of concern to the environmentalist, but also the resultant pollution of the biosphere. Dirty, choking skies claim victims of lung disease daily while acid rain tears down everything from buildings to ecosystems. In addition, the release of carbon dioxide feeds the process of global warming.

The fact is that many items transported long distances can be grown locally, but there is more and more a trend among large food stores to buy only out of centralized warehouses that have contracts with corporate farm conglomerates operating in distant states or even countries. To counter this, some movements have been started in an attempt to encourage support of local farmers' markets. Buying locally not only prevents unnecessary transport of these items, but also keeps the local environment green, both economically and physically, because it pays farmers to keep working their fields instead of selling them to developers or larger, mechanized farm companies.[22] Buying locally also provides freshly picked foods that are richer in nutrients than foods picked green and ripened artificially after transport.

Another positive action is the encouragement of city gardens of vegetables and fruit trees around private homes,

---

[22] Some governments have worked for a system of "transferable development rights," by which farmers can sell the housing rights to their land without actually giving up the land, allowing developers to build more densely elsewhere. A simplified explanation can be found in "Bountiful Broward: Going ... Going ... Almost Gone" from the Broward Soil and Water Conservation District • 6179 SW 45th St. • Suite 6173L • Ft. Lauderdale, FL 33314.

apartment buildings, and even in public parks. It seems absurd that city children are reduced to stealing fruit from the trees of conscientious home gardeners because neither municipal parks officials nor the children's parents provide a legitimate outlet for this very natural instinct to procure fresh produce.

A True Environmental Concern

In order for people to eat meat, eggs, or dairy products, livestock must be fed and housed and their products refrigerated, which requires a tremendous amount of resources. According to animal scientists at Ohio State University, the best animal production returns only about 35% of the fossil fuel energy invested, whereas the least efficient plant crop returns 328%.

One-third of all the raw materials consumed in the United States are used to produce our animal-based diet. Over half of the clean water used in this country goes to raising livestock; a total vegetarian can be fed using less than 10% of the water required to feed a meat-eater.

Approximately 90% of oats, 85% of corn, and 80% of soybeans grown in this country are fed to livestock. The food that could be saved if humans consumed plant foods directly would be enough to feed the starving people of the world many times over. According to the President's Science Advisory Committee, 15 people can be fed a vegetarian diet on the amount of land needed to produce a meat-centered diet for one person. The intensive farming techniques required to produce an animal-based diet have led to the loss of more than half of the original topsoil in the United States. Millions of acres of formerly productive and diverse tropical rainforest have been cleared and are now used to graze livestock; the consequences of this destruction are not yet known. Cows and cattle are the largest source of methane emissions, one of the most potent greenhouse gases.

In addition to the waste of resources inherent in raising and killing animals for food is the creation of waste. Any system that concentrates thousands of animals in a small area must deal with disposing huge amounts of excrement, much of which winds up choking off our waterways. The livestock industry is responsible for more water pollution in the United

The Most Noble Diet

States than all other industries combined.[23] Runoff from feedlots and slaughter-houses has contaminated water supplies across the nation. In a more spacious setting, animal wastes are natural fertilizers for the soil, but in great concentrations actually "burn" the soil, and it remains uneconomical to collect and ship these wastes somewhere else for distribution.

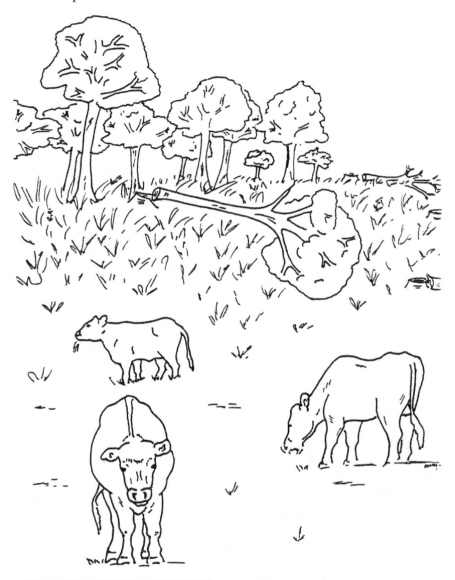

[23] See John Robbins, *Diet for a New America,* 1987, Stillpoint Pub., for a full treatment of this subject.

CHAPTER 5
POLITICS

The next nobler level of diet selection involves expressing political opinions through supporting or boycotting foods produced in a particular country or by a particular business enterprise. There are basically three ways that people express political opinions in their diet selection. The first is by buying the foods produced in a particular country they seek to support. An obvious example is buying foods produced in one's home country (such as "Buying American for a stronger America"), but, as will be discussed later, this has ramifications that go beyond political matters, when executed in a thoughtful manner. A more subtle example, though, of political support occurs in many of the ethnic neighborhoods of major cities throughout the world where products exported from the people's homeland are bought in large quantities, often at premium prices.

The second mode of political ideology being manifested through food selection is refusal to buy the produce of countries that are seen as the enemy. Many Jewish people, despite the recent peace treaty, would prefer not to buy items exported from the Arabic countries. Conversely, many Arabs would not buy Israeli exports. In a similar vein, people all across the United States have in the past refused to buy goods produced in the Soviet Union, especially after the Soviet government committed inhumane acts like invading Afghanistan or shooting down a South Korean airliner. Russian vodka and Russian caviar were two of the most visible items boycotted. Another example has been the refusal by many individuals and corporations to buy products from South Africa as a protest against the blatant racist policies of that government.

A third form of political expression is a boycott of products produced by a certain company or group of companies within an industry. Probably the most famous example of this in the

The Most Noble Diet

United States was in the 1960s when many Americans did not buy grapes and lettuce unless assured that those products were picked by the unionized farmworkers who were struggling for recognition at the time. The American people were touched by the wretched working conditions allowed to exist among many of the non-unionized harvesters of these crops. Indeed, many did without these food staples for quite a while, and when given a choice, paid more for the union-certified products.

One of that boycott's leaders, Cesar Chavez, tried again in the late 1980s to get Americans to stop buying table grapes. The goal this time was to get growers to stop using certain pesticides that were hazardous to the farm workers. The results of this latter boycott were much less dramatic, at least compared to the effects of Meryl Streep's campaign against the use of the chemical Alar on apples. The Alar issue was a matter of consumer's health, and in particular children's health. An example of a company boycotted in the United States because of their actions in other countries is the action against the Nestle Company. The central issue in this instance was the questionable marketing techniques used by the company to try to sell its infant formula to mothers in the poorer nations of the world. Dressing women in white and calling them "milk nurses" as promoters for their product, Nestle swayed many mothers into thinking formula was somehow medically recommended over breast-feeding. The results were disastrous. Because the poor women buying the formula often did not have sanitary water with which to mix the concoction, their babies frequently died from the diarrhea of the dysentery that followed. In addition, many of the families did not always have the money to buy as much formula as their babies needed. Well-meaning mothers would dilute the formula two or three times as much as recommended, and their babies subsequently suffered from undernourishment. Tragically, the mothers' breast milk dried up from disuse before it could be used as a supplement. In any event, it took Nestle several years to withdraw this advertising campaign. Meanwhile, many thousands of conscionable people in the more affluent countries were refusing to buy Nescafe coffee, Nestle's chocolate, and other items under the company's manufacture.

The precedent set by these instances of using our consumer dollars either to help or to protest a political cause is a promising one, especially for the theme of this book. Each of us can not only make a statement, but actually do our share to change things. Imagine how effective this could be if everyone participated. There is an almost universal feeling that any child born into this world deserves to have enough to eat. Although there is undoubtedly a lot of controversy over whether so many should be allowed to be born in the first place, only a callous person would approve of allowing children, already alive and breathing, to die by the millions from malnutrition or starvation. The goal of this book is to provide a means whereby all of us can do our share, merely by spending our consumer dollars where they do the most good, and equally important, not spending them where they perpetuate a horrendous situation.

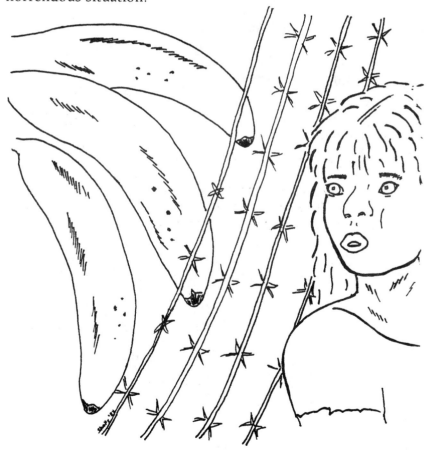

The Most Noble Diet

CHAPTER 6
NONVIOLENCE

To cause as little suffering as possible in one's life is the central precept of *Ahimsa* (nonviolence). This centuries-old practice was popularized in Western countries by the 1982 Academy Award-winning movie *Gandhi*, and increasing numbers of people are adopting this ethic into their life-style. Much of the Animal Liberation movement is a manifestation of this ethic.

In terms of food, the method of procurement can be used as the criteria for the relative appropriateness of consuming it. The nonviolence-oriented person considers the contrast between a freshly killed lamb and a freshly picked piece of fruit or vegetable, such as a tomato, strawberry, or watermelon. Cutting these "foods" open would reveal a similar color of red, but they would certainly differ in their overall sensory appeal. The inside of a fruit is generally appealing – pleasantly fragrant, delicately textured, and sweet tasting. On the other hand, the animal's "innards" contain rubbery-looking organs and greasy fat pockets amid a torrent of gushing blood, accompanied by the stench of death.

Whereas a true carnivore salivates at the sight of another animal freshly killed, the revulsion most human beings experience indicates our vegetarian inclination. The nonviolence-conscious person looks beyond the broiled and "dressed" lamb chop, "seasoned to taste," and sees the animal who suffered and died. Most of us seek to avoid this dark side of the meat industry, the full specter of violence and mutilation that went before, so it is by design that factory farms and slaughterhouses are usually unmarked windowless buildings in sparsely populated areas.

Some people state a belief that God put the animals on this earth to serve our purposes, to be killed and eaten. However, it would seem that only a cruel God would give the creatures of the world the ability to feel pain, the desire for pleasure, and an overwhelming urge to survive, if the animals' only purpose was to live their entire lives in cages and be slaughtered on an assembly line. It would seem that those who act with compassion toward all of creation are the ones acting most in accordance with God's wishes.

Others defend meat eating as natural. They state that animals kill one another, as if the actions of others can be an ethical excuse for their own actions. They also say that other animals are incapable of morality, and thus deserve no moral consideration. But there are many cases that tell us otherwise. For example, in an experiment conducted by humans, captive rhesus monkeys were fed only if they were willing to pull a chain and electrically shock an unrelated monkey whose agony was in plain view through a one-way mirror. Rather than inflicting suffering on another, these animals chose to go hungry, suffering for days, even weeks.[24]

Despite the fact that we and other animals are capable of morality and actions motivated by compassion, some defend killing and eating animals as "natural." Even if, at some point in history, taking an innocent life for food was "natural," there is nothing natural about the way animals are treated today.

Eco-hypocrisy

Preservation of high-profile endangered animal species is one ecological issue that has survived, at least until now, the onslaught of big business into environmentalism. This plays on deep emotion. Of *course* we love animals. We don't want to see the bison or the grey wolf become extinct, never to be seen again. What would *our* lives be then?

Despite our good intentions and our "love" of animals, this entire process is a facade for our own selfishness and greed. We have no concern for the *individual* animal behind the glass screen of the TV. We have no empathy for the *individual* animal living her entire life in a cage. What interests us is the level of novelty. Our money goes to ensure that the show will continue into the future, so we can "ooh" and "ahh" for the next human generation, living in the next layer of subdivisions built upon the habitat of creatures not fortunate enough to be "rare" or "cute." The animals we watch could be wind-up dolls for all

---

[24] Cited in *Shadows of Forgotten Ancestors,* Drs. Carl Sagan and Anne Druyan, Random House, 1992.

The Most Noble Diet

we care, as long as they are of different sizes and colors and act on command.

These species of animals with whom we concern ourselves so much that we cage them to "preserve" them are made up of individual sentient creatures – beings with feelings and desires separate from our view of them. An animal *feels* no differently, suffers no less, if it is the last of a species or one of billions. Our selfishness to maintain a menagerie for our aesthetic pleasure ignores the actual lives that exist separately from our "diversity" census.

The hypocrisy of our actions is overwhelming. We write a check for the preservation of the bison, then we consume the roasted flesh of domesticated cattle. We marvel at the beauty, grace, or humor of the hundreds of animals contained in a few blocks of a zoo in the middle of the city, but we fail to consider the sordid reality of the situation – that many animals died to bring just one to live an incarcerated and unnatural life for our caged convenience, while those left behind are killed by our expansion.

The very simple fact of the situation is that *every* animal – from the tiger in the wild to the baboon pacing in the cage to the rabbit shackled in the lab to the pig screaming as she is beaten to the slaughterhouse's killing floor – is endangered. Scientific labels such as species cannot change this. The ability to sense and suffer is not dependent on the number of similar others.

We wall ourselves away, divorced and set apart from the nature that brought us forth. Our "heritage" thus becomes a pool of resources for our use, or a list of Latin species names to be defended. Lost is something much greater – the spirit of nature that nurtures and defends *us*.

It is time to look upon the world and all it holds – from scenic vistas to overflowing landfills, from tropical rainforests to clear-cut timber stands, from the last of a certain flower to just one of billions of "food" animals – with respect, a respect separate from set, selfish desires of what the world should be for *us*.

The Transformation of Animals into Food

People often say, "As long as animals are raised and killed humanely, I don't have a problem eating them." In the high-volume livestock industry of today, driven solely by profit, animals are by no means raised or killed humanely.

Factory Farms. Animals used for food are explicitly excluded from anti-cruelty laws. Livestock have no protection from abuses that would be criminal offenses if done to pet or even stray dogs or cats.

In North America today, most animals do not live on traditional farms. To meet the demand for inexpensive meat, they are raised in intensive confinement systems, as though they are objects in a factory. In general, these systems crowd as many animals as can fit into one building, usually an inconspicuous, windowless shed.

The animals must live in their own excrement, from which high concentrations of ammonia burn their sinuses and cause respiratory diseases that have even been fatal to workers.[25] In order to keep them alive under these conditions, high doses of antibiotics are mixed with their feed: over 50% of all antibiotics used in this country are fed to livestock, a practice banned in the 1970s by the European Economic Community. Even so, 20–40% of pigs die before taken to slaughter.[26]

Hormones are mixed with the animals' feed and their environments are manipulated (more or less light, warmer or colder temperatures, altered feeding schedules) to make them grow faster, larger, and produce more than their skeletal systems can handle, causing pain in their overloaded and often extremely swollen joints. Living their entire lives, day after day, on concrete, cement, or wire increases these problems.

Animals in slaughterhouses can hear those ahead of them being shackled and killed, can smell the stench, and can sometimes see the slaughter. All animals fight for their lives and struggle with their remaining strength to get away.

---

[25] *Feedstuffs*, Dec. 31, 1984
[26] *Feedstuffs*, Jan. 30, 1989

The Most Noble Diet

Forget the pig is an animal.
Treat him just like a machine in a factory. [27]

Pigs. Over 80% of pigs in the U.S. are intensively confined. The stress of these crowded conditions can cause fighting and tail biting. To combat this, the young pigs have their tails cut off without anesthesia.

Breeding sows are constrained for their 16-week pregnancies in a gestation crate barely larger than their bodies. Their piglets are born on a slatted metal floors or concrete. The mothers are kept in a farrowing stall that does not allow them to move until their young are weaned.

Most pigs are taken to slaughter when less than a year old. By that time, 10–30% have gastric ulcers, 30–80% have lesions typical of pneumonia, and up to 90% have degenerative joint disease.[28] They are crammed onto trucks and sometimes ride for days to auction and then to slaughter, without food (and sometimes water), while being exposed to the weather. When the truck pulls up to the slaughterhouse, the pigs, sensing what lies ahead, must be forced off the truck with bruising blows and/or electric shocks. In the slaughterhouse, some pigs regain consciousness during slaughter, despite attempts at stunning.

Male Dairy Calves. To keep their flesh tender, most veal calves live their shortened lives confined in tiny stalls without room to move or turn around, in a windowless shed where the lights are turned on only for feeding. They are fed a diet deficient in iron so their flesh remains pale, and commonly have been known to lick and gnaw the bars of their cages trying to get iron. Up to 20% die before reaching slaughter age – 16 weeks.

Dairy Cows. Over 60% of dairy cows in the United States are intensively confined. They are repeatedly impregnated to continue their milk production. Their calves are taken from them within hours after birth, causing both mother and calf great distress. The demand for dairy products creates the veal market because male offspring are raised for veal.

---

[27] *Hog Farm Management*, Sept. 1976
[28] *Science*, June 16, 1989

The stress of continual pregnancy, combined with vacuum milk extraction, exacts a great physical toll. In 1960, the average cow produced 2.5 tons of milk per year; in 1990 she produced 7 tons. In 1993, the U.S. government approved Bovine Growth Hormone (BGH) (also known as Bovine Somatotropin – BST), which will make cows produce 20–40% more milk. In addition to further stressing the cows' joints (from carrying too much milk) and increasing the incidence of mastitis (infection and inflammation of the udder), industry tests indicate that BGH causes enlargement of internal organs and increased intolerance to heat.

Dairy cows can be electrically shocked by "stray voltage" while on milking machines. Some dairy farmers report some cows becoming so distressed at the sight of the machines that they defecate or urinate out of fear.

Each dairy cow is impregnated every year ("freshened," as the industry calls it) and her calf taken away soon after birth to keep the milk flowing. Although they can live 25 years under normal conditions, modern dairy cows are slaughtered after five years of constant production.

Laying Hens. Over 95% of egg-laying hens in the United States are intensively confined. Typically, four or five hens live in a cage with a wire floor about the size of a folded newspaper. Chickens have been discovered "literally grown fast to the cage ... the flesh of the toes grew completely around the wire."[29] Layers of these cages are stacked one on top of the other. The hens are at the mercy of automated feeding and watering systems, which sometimes malfunction. The daily collection of the dead is not yet automated; about 25% die before being taken to slaughter.

The stress from cramped conditions leads to the birds attacking one another. To combat this, the farmers cut off a portion of the birds' beaks without anesthesia, using a hot knife or a guillotine-like device. In a report commissioned by the British Parliament, Professor F. W. Brambell noted that "between the horn and the bone is a thin layer of highly sensitive soft tissue ... debeaking cuts through this complex of the horn, bone, and sensitive tissue, causing severe pain."

---

[29] *Poultry Tribune*, Feb. 1974

Sometimes, the birds' toes are removed just behind the claw, also without anesthesia.

Small birds, producing eggs too large for their bodies, sometimes have their uterus prolapse – that is, expelled along with the egg. Besides the obvious pain, this can also lead to cannibalism, as the other birds attack the pink/red uterine wall.

When production slows, the birds in some operations are force molted to renew their laying. This is done by giving them no food for 1–2 weeks. This forced molting, which can be done several times during their lives, impairs their immune system, increasing Salmonella contamination of their eggs.

Egg-laying hatcheries don't have any use for male chicks. These hatchlings are discarded and die from suffocation, gassing, drowning, or being ground up alive. They are then put into pet food or used as fertilizer.

Chicken and Turkey. Over 99% of poultry in the United States are intensively confined. Thousands or tens of thousands of birds live in one building with little room to move around. They are debeaked, and sometimes declawed, without anesthesia.

Like all intensively confined animals, these birds are subject to heat stress. For example, 300,000 broiler chickens died from heat stress on June 9, 1993 in Delaware, Maryland, and Virginia.

Many slaughterhouses do not bother to stun birds before cutting their throats. In those that attempt to stun them, the birds are hung from a conveyor belt and often lift their heads, missing the stunning tank. Others regain consciousness after having their throat cut. Sometimes a bird will break free and be left to die thrashing in pools of blood on the killing floor. Other birds who do not bleed to death are boiled alive in the scalding tank.

Cattle. Cattle spend half their lives in crowded feedlots. Some are painfully branded with hot irons and castrated and dehorned without anesthesia. They are slaughtered in two ways:

Stunning (captive bolt pistol) – Trying to shoot terrified, struggling animals is difficult, and the bolt often misses the mark, injuring them without rendering them unconscious. They are shackled by one leg, hoisted upside down (which can break bones, dislocate joints, and tear muscles, tendons, and ligaments), and their throats are cut. Some stunned cows regain consciousness before bleeding to death.

Kosher – This method requires the animals to be fully conscious when their throats are cut and while they bleed to death. Much non-Kosher meat comes from animals killed by Kosher slaughter methods.

Transport. During transport, animals are commonly not fed or given water for up to three days. They are packed tightly together to minimize costs, living in each other's excrement, and are exposed to extreme weather conditions in the open trucks and rail cars. Pigs have arrived at the slaughterhouse frozen to the side of the truck. Shipping fever, which can be fatal, is common in cattle transported long distances to the feedlot, then to the stockyards, and then to the slaughterhouse.

Baby chicks are sometimes shipped by the U.S. Postal Service. These trips can take three days, with 20% dying en route.

Downers. The trauma of being raised in intensive confinement systems – coupled with exposure to extreme weather and the lack of food, water, and veterinary care during transport – can result in animals, usually dairy cows and breeding sows, being too sick or weak to walk, even when beaten or shocked with electric prods. They are often dragged by chains to slaughter. Handlers also tie animals to a stationary objects and drive the trucks out from underneath them, often resulting in broken limbs. Sometimes downed animals are left to starve to death.

Industry Attitudes. In a letter to *Farmer and Stockbreeder*, a veterinarian wrote, "I hope many of my colleagues will join me in saying that we are already tolerating systems of husbandry which, to say the least of it, are downright cruel.... Cost effectiveness and conversion ratios are all very well in a robot state; but if this is the future, then the sooner I give up both farming and farm veterinary work as well the better."[30]

Animal handlers often react toward the animals with impatience and sometimes blatant cruelty. In the trade

---

[30] Cited in *Animal Factories*, Jim Mason and Peter Singer, Harmony Books, 1990.

The Most Noble Diet

magazine *Meat and Poultry*, livestock consultant Temple Grandin reported numerous cases of "deliberate cruelty", including workers taking "sadistic pleasure from shooting the eyes out of cattle," bashing the heads of cattle with the headgate of a hydraulic shoot and electrically shocking animals in sensitive areas of their bodies.

Grandin says, "[It is] easier to maintain a good attitude in plants with a slower line speed. ... The constant pressure to keep up with the line leads to abuse." In spite of this, the average U.S. slaughterhouse line accelerated 22% during the 1980s.

The National Turkey Federation opposes humane poultry slaughter legislation because "it would subject turkey processors to a potentially expensive new set of regulations when no one has demonstrated a problem with the existing slaughter process."[31] The Animal Welfare Committee of the American Veterinary Medical Association says that laying hens' "low economic value makes it difficult to justify costly new slaughter techniques."

Paté de Fois Grâs. Paté (ground liver) comes from ducks or geese who have a metal pipe shoved down their throats three times a day and have massive amounts of food forced into their stomachs in order to enlarge their livers. Sometimes their stomachs burst from this procedure.

Fish. Neurological evidence indicates that fish feel pain when they are hooked and when they suffocate. In addition, the driftnets used to catch most fish can be up to 35 miles long. Dolphins, whales, birds, and sea turtles are drowned when they swim in the paths of these nets.

Many areas of the ocean have been stripped clean because of overfishing. Animals such as sea lions who compete with people for fish are shot or fed fish packed with explosives. All non-target species, often the majority of the catch, are thrown back dead. Larry Cotter, a fisheries consultant for the National Marine Fisheries Service has called the waste "a national scandal and an unconscionable disgrace."

---

[31] *Turkey World*, Apr./May 1993

Beyond Might Makes Right

The environmentalist is concerned with not upsetting the balance of nature as a whole, for we are all part of the environment, and to harm the environment is to harm ourselves. The politically minded person is concerned with keeping a fair balance of power. These, along with personal health and pleasure, are all largely self-centered concerns, whereas the compassion for all life – from a stranger on the street to the last blue whale to one tiny chick – is a higher level of consciousness and nobility. It incorporates all of the other concerns and applies them beyond ourselves.

It is not as though we are unable to turn away from the suffering of others. There is no personal physical discomfort, no political take-over, no holocaust, no catastrophe to be feared. It can be out of sight, out of mind: the death of one animal passes and we continue our lives unchanged, unthinking, and uncaring. The philosophy of nonviolence, which teaches that positive, joyful feelings can result from feeling responsible for preventing unnecessary suffering, is the greatest expression of our morality: to express concern for the individual well-being of all sentient beings – creatures capable of suffering.

But What About Plants?

A typical retort against a person who follows the precepts of nonviolence is "How far will you go?" People constantly confront vegetarians with "Plants feel pain, too," attempting to use *reducto ad absurdum* as a defense of eating animals.

In his book *Erehwon*, Samuel Butler wrote about a mythical country where the government, in its effort to promote nonviolence, eventually outlawed the eating of everything except the fruits that fell from the trees of their own accord. Because the citizens were not very turned on by the prospect of rotting fruit for every meal, a black market of immense proportion soon arose where one could purchase everything from green tomatoes to butchered lambs. It was not long before everyone, including the highest government officials, bought their food illegally, and the laws concerning food consumption became the society's jokes (just as those laws in some parts of this country that forbid now common practices like premarital sex).

The Most Noble Diet

The lessons of this are twofold. First, of course, it is senseless to attempt to legislate morality. The morals of a society usually reflect the current thinking of the mass of people, and popular opinion slowly changes over time. Just as it is generally acceptable and legal to exploit and kill other animals for any reason today, it was once generally acceptable and legal to exploit less powerful humans, be they of a different skin color, gender, or religion. Even today, anti-gay-rights legislation is popular in many areas. Institutions such as the press publicize "different" behavior, such as using dogs for food or granting medical insurance to same-sex spouses, and the public voices either support or outrage. There is no law, for instance, against eating dogs in this country, yet when the Los Angeles animal shelter planned to send pound dogs scheduled for execution to Thailand to be eaten, there was such an outrage that the plan was halted (and the dogs destroyed and discarded).

Second, when one is dealing with philosophies such as nonviolence, there must be a reasonable understanding to temper extremes, lest unworkable conclusions be reached and the entire principle be discarded. Under the tenets of nonviolence, our senses and innate compassion constitute an appropriate guide.

Think of the smell and sight of a field of newly mown hay or grass. Is that the stench of death, the cry of pain and agony (perhaps the latter, if you have hay fever!)? We may associate a sense of loss when a grand old tree is felled to make way for a new shopping mall, even more so if it happens to be the old apple tree you and the other neighborhood kids used to climb and pick a tasty treat. It is humane to like and respect trees, but it is probably unreasonable to be afraid of picking their fruit for fear of harming them. When a plant is being trimmed, we have no innate sense of suffering occurring; we experience no discomfort or unease at the sight a field of corn being harvested.

Science supports our intuition. There is no biological evidence to indicate that plants suffer. They do not possess any semblance of a central nervous system to process stimuli, no thalamus to produce hormones that create the emotions of pain or fear. Furthermore, pain would serve no purpose for plants; because they have no capacity to escape from threats, any energy and resources invested in sensing pain would be lost.

However, if one is concerned with the taking of any life, a vegetarian diet requires many fewer plants to feed a person because it avoids the inefficient step of feeding plants to other animals first. In addition, much of a vegetarian diet comes from foods that do not require killing a living plant – fruits, seeds, nuts, beans, and grains are harvested following senescence. It is not necessary to kill plants to eat of their bounty.

A Nonviolent Diet?

Few ethical people would disagree that vegetarianism is the direction to take, but to what extent? There are many types of people who call themselves vegetarians, from those who eat only certain types of animal flesh (or eat meat only occasionally), to those who eat no products derived from animals at all. The latter believe that theirs is the only harmless diet.

Not abstaining from meat but still calling oneself a vegetarian is akin to being a perfect Christian but believing in God occasionally and only following the precepts of their religion only when convenient. It is difficult to consider this person a true Christian because this person demeans Christianity and treats God as a matter of convenience.

The same is true for periodic meat-eaters: they ignore the basic principles of vegetarianism and still view animals as nothing but food – sentient beings whose purpose is to produce flesh for human convenience and taste. So long as there is still the demand for the corpses of animals for food, there will be someone called upon to do the killing.

Many people call themselves vegetarians because they eat no "red" meat,[32] having given up the flesh of cows, sheep, and pigs, while continuing to eat (probably more than previously) the flesh of turkeys, chicken, and fish. The euphemism of "red" meat somehow implies that birds and fish do not bleed, or have white instead of red blood.

Although there may generally be less fat in the meat of these animals than in the larger mammals, there is still no proven health advantage gained from eating any kind of meat. When was the last news report that found a disease linked to

---

[32] Animal flesh is generally prepared or dyed to look red because it is naturally a very unappetizing brown.

vegetarianism instead of to consumption of meat? All flesh foods have about the same amount of cholesterol, and lower-fat flesh has more cholesterol per calorie. They also have an excessive protein content.

From the point of view of nonviolence, it actually engenders more killing when a switch is made to these so-called "white" meats, because the smaller size of birds and fish necessitates butchering more individual animals to produce the same number of meals. The vast number of poultry consumed has created intensive and extremely cruel conditions. Many people consume a whole chicken or a whole fish at one sitting, whereas a dead cow can feed a family for several weeks.

There are some who would argue that birds and fish represent "lower" life forms than our fellow mammals, the pigs and cows. However, suffering is suffering regardless of our hierarchy of life; anyone who has heard a chicken fight the knife and scream when being butchered could not reasonably doubt that it was suffering horribly. The screams of birds are simply different from those of mammals, not less authentic.

Fish, who cannot scream, express their agony through body language, as a human mute may. It has been found that the skin of a fish, which acts as a sensory organ for life in the water, contains nerve sensitivity very similar to the human eye. Thus, the frenzied, desperate slapping of a hundred fish dumped on the deck of a ship is as if a hundred eyes were being repeatedly poked with wooden sticks.

Most birds can fly and most fish can swim in ways we can only robotically mimic with sophisticated machinery. Certainly, no group of birds or fish has developed, or even desired, the elaborate means of enslaving, exploiting, and exterminating others. In many ways, it is we who are the "lower" animals.

Some argue that we have inherently less compassion for beings who are very different from ourselves. If this were true, why are we so drawn to these animals, gazing in wonder at the varied birds at the aviary? Why do so many people buy aquariums to watch the grace and beauty of living fish? It is not in the interests of the confined animals to live that way, but rather for the convenience of human beings who wish to enjoy observing them. Is it not perverse to kill and eat that which provides us so much pleasure?

The Most Noble Diet •42•

It is in life that animals appeal to our curiosity, our awe. If we were to see an animal in pain, a bird with a broken wing, a rabbit hit by a car, we feel sympathy and want to help, even if just having eaten the animal's kin for our dinner.

We may resist compassion, but it is a part of us.

Lacto-Ovo Vegetarianism.

The most prevalent form of true vegetarianism in the United States today (and this may be changing) is lacto-ovo vegetarianism, the practice of eating no meat of any kind but still consuming dairy products (milk, cheese, yogurt, etc.) and eggs in addition to plant-derived foods. This is the logical first step into vegetarianism because food like cheese and eggs have similar characteristics to flesh-foods (high in fat, very filling), and yet do not overtly involve killing.[33] I emphasize "overtly" because in today's commercial setting, the indirect result of demand for dairy and eggs is greater suffering, as described previously. The dairy farms and egg factories are merely stopping points on the way to the slaughterhouse.

The Vegan Alternative.

As discussed previously, dairy cows must be impregnated repeatedly during their lives to keep their milk production flowing. The resulting calves are, of course, in competition with humans for the milk, so these young beings are whisked away immediately after birth. The males are taken to the veal pens – torture chambers in which the calves are kept in complete darkness, unable to move. In a few months, they are butchered

The female calves are allowed to mature to take their mothers' places. As the Moms reach what would normally be one-third of their normal life span, their milk production falls off. Instead of being sent to pasture as a reward for providing our children with her milk, she is sent to the slaughterhouse to become low-grade beef.

This is not the way it has to be, but it is the way it always will be in the present system, where profits are paramount and animals are granted no consideration. Our demand for dairy products creates an industry that, in order to be competitive, keeps its costs as low as possible. This means no extra feed or

---

[33] Although most cheese contains rennet, a slaughter-derived product.

freedom for unwanted babies (calves), nor any reprieve for the retired workers (milked-out mothers)

Chickens kept for egg production are in similar binds. Four to five hens are crammed into one of thousands of cages stacked in a single building. According to *Poultry Digest*, the typical flock size in one building is 80,000.[34] The birds' environment and feeding schedule are manipulated to maximize their egg laying. Whereas a free chicken would build a nest and separate herself from the flock to lay her eggs, these caged hens are hardly even able to cower in the corner of the wire cage, and their eggs immediately roll across the sloped mesh floor and eventually then off to market.

This stress causes the birds, who normally have a social order within their flocks, to attack one another. The solution might seem to be less crowded cages, and though this may be more humane, it is not profit-maximizing. To maintain the same number of birds while allowing for the survival of those that would otherwise be pecked to death, the farmers debeak the birds. They can't attack each other, but they are still under the same maddening conditions. Sometimes Nature, in her mercy, allows the beaks to grow back slowly, but humans, in our lack of mercy, debeak the hens again.

These tortured animals are only allowed to live about 18 months, rather than their normal 15-year life span, but sometimes not before they suffer a final indignity – forced molting, which is designed to stimulate a last round of egg production. After being subjected to bright lights for up to 17 hours a day, the lights are turned off and food and water removed for two days. After the forced molting, the hens who survive may be productive enough to keep around for a few more months. Once the statistics for the entire building are no longer sufficient, the entire lot is shipped to slaughter to become soup. Like other animals on their way to our plates, they are not fed the last days of their horrible lives, for the food would be "wasted" – not sufficiently converted to fat and muscle.[35]

---

[34] July, 1978

[35] It was this practice that led to Animal Liberation Action's First Annual Fast for Farm Animals, where activists fasted for three days outside of a Cincinnati slaughterhouse.

How are the layers replaced? Batches of eggs are incubated – artificially, of course, because no hen is allowed the time or space to sit on the eggs, or perform any other natural acts. As soon as the batch of chicks hatch, they are placed on a huge conveyor belt, with the "healthy-looking" females plucked off and taken to a crowded pen until they are mature enough to be debeaked and replace Mom in the tiny cage.

The rest of the fuzzy little chicks are left on the conveyor belt until they fall off the end of the line. Here they are gassed, drowned, or merely left to suffocate under the weight of the other chicks. They are then crushed into cat food or fertilizer.

This is the modern picture of the dairy and egg industries, hidden from the public as carefully as animal slaughter: every glass of milk, cheese pizza, or egg-over-easy comes from confined, tormented females whose miserable lives are ended once their productivity no longer maximizes profits. Her manipulated and mangled body is then dismembered and served to us as the final insult.

Responsibility for these deaths ought to taint the taste of omelets, cheese soufflés, and milkshakes for every consumer with a conscience.

Vegans, or "pure" vegetarians, generally believe that we as ethical human beings have no right to kill or harm other animals unnecessarily. Thus, vegans are the epitome of nonviolence in their dietary practice. Just as we recognize the rights of other human beings of a different nationality, race, gender, intelligence level, or sexual preference to live free of exploitation, vegans maintain that all sentient beings should be allowed to live without exploitation.

There is no characteristic that separates every human being from all non-human animals. The continual search for a unique attribute led psychologist Paul Chance to conclude that we are "the only creature on Earth that tries to prove that it is different from, and preferably superior to, other species."[36]

Indeed, characteristics such as intelligence, awareness, and altruism exist in a continuum, with individuals from other species having a greater capacity for these abilities than some humans. Even so, these criteria should not matter in our

---

[36] *Psychology Today*, Jan. 1988

The Most Noble Diet

interactions with others. As Jeremy Bentham, nineteenth-century Professor of Jurisprudence at Oxford University said, "The question is not, 'Can they reason?' nor, 'Can they talk?' But rather, 'Can they suffer?'"

Although the human species obviously has the might to claim superiority over the rest of the animal kingdom, our ability to inflict suffering and exploit the weaker for our own benefit does not make it morally right. Would we follow the same diet if each one of us had to slash the throat of an animal we knew, whom we had raised from birth? Should we feel comfortable paying others to do the killing so we do not have to see it or think about it?

Vegans are often accused of being naive to the fact that life is cruel and that other animals kill in nature. (There is nothing "natural" about a factory farm, however.) But the truly superior human beings have always based their actions on compassion for all. As moral beings, it is possible, even imperative, for us to live without intentionally contributing to the suffering of the animals with whom we share the world. Justice demands no less.

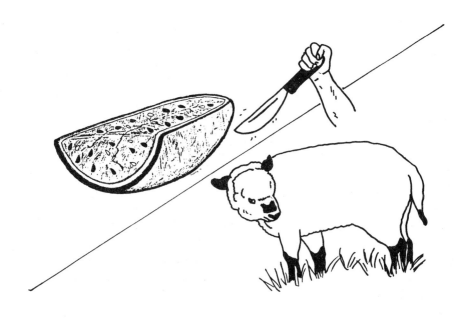

CHAPTER 7
HUMANITY

The final level of consciousness in food selection is consideration of other human beings. As children, we are often taught to be wary of strangers; as adolescents, participation in sports or academic competitions means wanting to inflict a loss on the other team; as adults in the business world, it is often cut-throat economics – "dog eat dog" – to survive financially. We have to overcome these teachings to really feel for others, especially when those others are sociologically, culturally, and/or economically detached from us.

When appeals are made to help the hungry in distant lands, it is no accident that the faces of children are featured. We are much less distrusting of children of another culture than we are of adults, presumably because the cultural identity of a child is less formed. Toddlers don't speak very much, making themselves understood through expressions that are universal. As people grow up, however, they learn the language and customs of their land, becoming different – alien – from us.

It seems to be almost part of human nature to try to divide groups into smaller groups, in an attempt to make our individual group seem more important and superior to the rest. Many people continually divide the world by random and impertinent traits into ever-decreasing circles of increasing similarity. As U.S. citizens, we are taught to take pride in being "Americans" (as though Canadians and Mexicans and everyone in Central and Southern America were part of a different, inferior continent). Yet taking pride in being a citizen of the country in which one was born is like taking pride in being white, or male, or tall. How can a characteristic conferred randomly upon an individual be a reason for egoism, for identifying and defending a certain group of people against some who are slightly different?

Countries are often considered to be in economic competition with each other. How many times do people object to foreign aid by saying, "Why don't we help our own first?" as though people living near us within some invisible boundary suffer more than others who are not "our own." On the other hand, the question can be asked, why do we allow other countries to sell us their food, when "their own" are much worse off?

The overfed countries of the world, while having some hungry in their midst, nevertheless waste an incredible amount of food. The greatest tragedy is where some of that food was originally grown.

The stereotyped doting mother's line, "Clean your plate, there are children starving in Africa" (or China, or Europe, depending on the decade) was the right idea, just incomplete in its execution. But rather than being the wise guy and telling mom to ship the leftovers overseas, what may really have done some good would have been to ask her to buy a little less at the store next time and just serve smaller portions.

The basic law of economics is the relationship between supply and demand. The more people buy of something (demand), the more the producers will market it (supply). If there is not enough of something for everyone, the people with the greatest buying power (money) will get the first package. In many cases, hunger is not created from a lack of potential for adequate production. Rather, the good land is often used for purposes other than growing sustenance food, because the wealthy land owners want to get the highest return from their property, even if that means there will be too little food for the poorest people.

What is being done with the land? The fields that once grew food crops in many of the poorer countries of the world are now used either to grow feed for animals, so that the wealthiest may eat meat, or to grow cash crops for export. These cash crops include non-edible items such as cotton and rubber, non-nutritious foods such as coffee, tea, cocoa, and sugar, and such non-staple food items such as bananas and pineapples. These items are shipped to wealthier countries because more money can be obtained for them than would be obtained if staple foods were grown and sold locally. The costs of these items are still low by the standards in the wealthy nations, though, because the laborers are paid far less than the U.S. minimum wage.

The Disappearing American Family Farm

This situation also forces many family farms in the United States out of business because they cannot hire workers at such a pittance. Unable to compete, these farmers are ultimately forced to sell their lands to corporations who reduce costs by grand-scale mechanization. In *Trading the Future,* authors James Wessel and Mort Hantman point out that two-thirds of farm income in the United States is received by 1% of "farmers" – in actuality, major corporations. (This also often leads to environmental degradation because the corporations generally care only about this year's profits; if there is no soil left next year, they can write off the loss and move to another area.)

These corporations often turn out inferior products, such as hard, greenish tomatoes that are easier to pick by machine. They are able to sell their products by undercutting the price of smaller farmers as well as by having exclusive contracts with supermarkets and restaurant chains, who are often part of the same parent corporation.

What We Can Do

If we were to stop buying imported food and other agricultural products, the demand would be reduced, forcing the producers in those countries to look to the native population for a market. What they would find would be an underpaid, underfed group of families who would buy all the food the land could produce, provided it was sold at a reasonable price relative to the average wages.

If we insist on buying locally produced and high-quality fresh produce, we will keep our local farm economy strong. If this produce costs a bit more, it would be well worth it in return for a sounder economy, a more sustainable relationship with the environment, better nutrition, and superior taste.

Scope of the Problem: Hungry Countries

Table 7-1 shows the average proportion of required calories available to people in several countries around the world. The three columns contain the figures over time to show the trend.

Table 7-1
Proportion of Required Daily Caloric Intake per Person

Country	1970	1980	1990
Ethiopia	87	74	70
Haiti	83	83	81
Kenya	98	89	83
Panama	108	99	97
Peru	108	99	96
France	134	135	141
United States	131	138	150

Source: Food and Agriculture Organization
        of the United Nations.
The State of Food and Agriculture, 1981, pp. 172-173;
FAO Production Yearbook, 1991, pp. 37-38.

It should be quite obvious which are the hungry countries and which are the well-fed or overfed ones. Ethiopia, for instance, is a hungry country because the people who live there could obtain, on average, only 87% of their food requirement in 1970, and this declined to only 70% in 1990. In stark contrast, every woman, man, and child in the United States, on average (which includes those going hungry), received 131% of their required daily caloric intake in 1970, and this increased to 150% by 1990, more than twice the intake of the people who live in Ethiopia! No wonder that the people in the United States collectively spend billions of dollars trying to lose weight.

While North American and European countries get fatter and fatter, the rest of the world gets hungrier. During the period covered in Table 7-1, tens of millions of people died of malnutrition and the accompanying diseases. The majority of those dying were children.

One may think that the hungry countries devote their national resources toward feeding their own people and that starvation is caused by unavoidable situations. However, for reasons previously discussed and shown in Tables 7-2 and 7-3, these countries are actually growing less food for their own people, instead using the land to produce crops for export.

Table 7-2
Cereal Production (thousands of hectares harvested)

Country	1970	1980	1990
Ethiopia	5217	5180	5190
Haiti	483	455	330
Kenya	1817	1631	1967
Panama	182	172	170
Peru	852	821	745
France	9413	9886	9328
United States	60,715	61,523	62,058

Source: Food and Agriculture Organization of the United Nations.
FAO Production Yearbook, 1981, 1991.

Countries that justify additional cash crops as a way to boost their national welfare are either misguided or just lying outright. Judging from the worsening conditions of nutrition as evidenced in Table 7-1, it is obvious that the strategy of trying to help the situation by increasing revenue (at the cost of land to produce food for national consumption) simply doesn't work. The money we spend in the United States for these cash crops never gets back to the workers, but remains in the hands of the rich land owners, multi-national conglomerates, and government tax collectors.

Table 7-2 shows what is happening to farm land used to grow cereals (wheat, corn, rice, etc.), the staple foods of poor people (and from a health standpoint, what should be the staple foods of everyone). Most hungry countries have actually decreased their land area planted in cereal crops between the years 1970 and 1990. In contrast, the well-fed countries have in some cases increased production land area; although these crops are not fed to people, but rather "cycled" through animals at about 10% efficiency (90% of the calories are expended converting the grains to flesh). In addition, these wealthy countries are able to buy food from other countries.

As shown by the drop in caloric intake per person in Table 7-1, it is disastrous when hungry countries decrease their cereal harvest. Imagine a country where the people are already hungry, the population is increasing (in spite of, and indirectly because of, all the children who starve to death daily), and yet the farmers are allowed, even encouraged, to grow less food for the people. This is mainly our fault for providing a market for other goods which makes abandoning staple crops more financially profitable.

Table 7-3
Selected Cash Crop Productions (in thousands of hectares harvested)

	1970	1980	1990
Coffee			
Haiti	30	34	34
Kenya	85	120	150
Panama	21	24	25
Peru	119	140	164
France	0	0	0
United States	1	1	1
Sugar Cane			
Ethiopia		11	15
Kenya		38	49
Peru		58	62
Cocoa			
Haiti	1	2	2
Peru	4	9	21
Tea			
Kenya	30	62	91
Peru	3	3	4
Bananas*			
Ethiopia	53	73	79
Kenya	111	135	210
Haiti	160	200	220
Panama	1007	1050	1170

* Banana production in thousands of metric tons
Source: Food and Agriculture Organization of the United Nations.
FAO Production Yearbook, 1981, 1991.

The Most Noble Diet   •52•

Table 7-3 shows the increases in land area devoted to several cash crops in hungry countries. It may or may not be exactly the same land that previously grew grain (or it may be cleared rainforest), but it is now producing coffee, tea, bananas, etc. The trend is unmistakable: the more products a country grows for export, the less food produced for the country's citizens.

One example is Kenya, a former British colony in eastern Africa, that was approaching (98%) fully providing its citizens in 1970 with their required daily caloric intake. Twenty years later, however, this figure had been reduced to 83%. During the same period, land area for cereal crops increased some, but not as fast as the population grew. However, during this period, area devoted to cash crops nearly doubled.

In 1990, as a result of ongoing famines and civil unrest, Kenya's neighbor to the north, Ethiopia, could provide its citizens with only 70% of the food needed daily, compared with 87% in 1970. However, the land devoted to staples decreased, while land devoted to cash crops increased during that period.

Coming a bit closer to home, Peru, on the west coast of South America, experienced a decline from 108% of caloric requirement in 1970 to 96% in 1990. Because 96% is so close to 100%, this might seem insignificant, but note that for the United States, the figures went from 131% in 1970 to 150% in 1990, and we still have hungry and malnourished people here. Thus, overfed people who eat well over 100% of their needs can make these averages artificially inflated. Don't be fooled into thinking that a population such as Peru's is almost fully fed at 96%; there are undoubtedly overfed people there eating well over 100% of their needs. As Tables 7-2 and 7-3 show, however, since the 1970s, Peru has reduced cereal crop area from 852,000 hectares to 745,000 hectares, a decline of about 17%. At the same time, coffee production area was increased by 28% from 1970 to 1990. Cocoa bean production, a small industry in 1970, increased 81% by 1990. Tea production increased relatively little in the same period.

It is worth dwelling upon the notion that even holding land in a constant amount for cash crops is unethical in the face of an increasingly hungry population. It's like a man being diagnosed as having lung cancer and saying he will not increase his smoking any further, just hold it at the same three packs a day he's been smoking for years. Like a cigarette machine in a cancer ward, cash crops have no place in a hungry country until the hunger there is completely eradicated.

Consider that Panama, in troubled Central America, went from 108% in 1970 of caloric intake per person to 97% in 1990, with 12,000 hectares being taken out of cereal crops production. In the same period, coffee acreage increased by 19%. As for its chief cash crop, Panama now grows enough bananas so that every child, woman, and man in the country could eat over six pounds of bananas every day,[37] if the bananas remained in the country.

In a feature article that appeared in the *Miami Herald* during September 1984, the "Brazilian Nut Wars" were meticulously documented. The story related the predicament of subsistence farmers who were trying to grow food for their families on land claimed by wealthy Brazil nut tree plantation owners. The latter were hiring groups of thugs to burn out and sometimes even kill the farmers and their families so the plantations could expand to meet export demands. Local priests who sided with the peasant farmers were also targeted with violence. All this, ironically, was done in the name of being able to sell more Brazil nuts to countries such as the United States, whose peak demand is at Christmas, the time supposedly for giving and goodwill toward all.

Roots of the Problem

Many of these hungry countries were taken over as colonies by European powers in the last century. At that time, these were self-sufficient tribal societies with relatively small populations. As the colonizers grabbed all the best farmlands to start plantations of cash crops for sale back home, the native peoples had less and less land for themselves. They started growing ill from malnourishment, with many of their children dying from its effects.

It has been shown that this type of situation helps bring on overpopulation, because families fearing loss of children from disease will have as many offspring as possible. It has been estimated that when malnutrition is rampant, a family has to have six children to be reasonably sure that at least one male

---

[37] Although not a very balanced diet, this would nevertheless represent over 100% of daily caloric needs.

child will survive to adulthood. As the standard of living increases, the birth rate generally decreases. This means that the world would not be "overrun" by poor people if we let them have enough food to be nourished properly and to ensure that their children survive. It actually contributes to the overpopulation problem when we buy these cash crop products and keep making the poor even poorer.

Being an Activist

In addition to removing from our diet luxury foods that come at the cost of subsistence crops of hungry people, we can help to speak on behalf of those being abused by the system. Share these ideas with your grocer, supermarket managers, and even restaurateurs. Request that they at least tone down their advertising of imported food items like bananas, coffee, tea, and out-of-season produce. Demand more local produce on display.

If that fails, go to the countryside and talk to the farmers themselves. Tell them you want to buy directly from them, at full retail price. Talk to your neighbors and organize a buying group to share the transportation time and expense. It can be a fun trip: fresh air, natural scenery, and an opportunity for healthful exercise in picking the harvest, loading the haul, etc. Many farmers have indoor growing facilities, such as greenhouses, or would be willing to build some if they knew that they had a sure market for off-season produce. In addition, some crops such as potatoes can be left in the ground during the winter and harvested as needed. Consider how comforting it would be to personally know your food processor, someone who would never intentionally put harmful additives on your plate, as opposed to the current system now, for which the government acts as the only watchdog.

Growing your own garden, outside if you have the space or can use public land, or inside in pots and window boxes, is the best way to provide maximum control over your own diet. It has been estimated (probably by corporate giants) that, considering all the time put into a home garden, the money saved over store-bought produce amounts to your having worked for a mere 25 cents an hour. Look on the bright side: you get the freshest, least adulterated food possible, good exercise, and a bonus of a quarter an hour!

Conclusion

In all ethical societies, gluttony is frowned upon. The type of gluttony referred to in this chapter is not merely excessive eating, but rather demanding a range of items that this world can supply only at a cost of poverty, malnutrition, or starvation deaths of others. Because we can actually have a better diet in all of the aspects discussed in this book, including better taste, health, and environment, there is no justification to continue to exploit the weaker and less fortunate beings with whom we share the Earth.

The 1970s brought a barrage of books by psychologist/authors on self-help or improving your self-image. The theme of those books was often that it was "all right" to be selfish, to consider yourself solely, and not to worry about the feelings or well-being of others around you. For individuals given to self-degradation, this is an important concept for coping with the stresses of life, but there is more to self-esteem and personal worth than being concerned only with immediate self-gratification.

The principles of this book do not contradict the self-help ideas. Rather, in the truest sense of self-esteem, pursuing the Most Noble Diet reinforces these concepts. By following the sequence of increasing consciousness in food selection (as well as in other daily decisions), an individual can feel the mastery of life returning to its proper place.

Many people experience a great helplessness about the problems and injustices in the world, feeling impotent, guilty, even deprived of power or control. By living a more Noble life, we can experience the joy of knowing we are doing our part in building a better world, a better community, a better environment, and a better self. Loving through this Nobility, the good that it does, and the injustices that it relieves, is indeed the greatest and broadest love of all. Only when we choose to shape our own destinies, by solving our problems through changing our behavior, can we ensure everlasting freedom for all.

Justice begins with us.

APPENDICES

The Most Noble Diet

APPENDIX A
A NOBLE DIET GUIDELINE

The chapters of this book discuss the principles of a Noble diet: eating, whenever obtainable, fresh, locally produced plant-derived foods without unnecessary additives or residues. It would be impossible to print one exact diet that would apply to all people at all locations at all times of year.

Table A-2 provides a listing of most of the usually consumed foods produced in the United States, as well as some unusual ones. However, it is each individual's task to determine appropriate selections, given their situation. What is provided here is a scheme to ensure nutritional adequacy on this type of diet.

How Much to Eat

The best determinant of how much to eat is your own appetite, provided that it is working right and if there are not too many seductive temptations by refined foods. No one knows better than you whether or not your weight is appropriate for your body height and frame. Muscle weighs more than fat, so an exercise program that increases your muscle mass may actually increase your weight, even though you appear slimmer. True measures of fat are determined by measuring fat-folds under the skin and/or by determining the percentage of your body weight that is fat (accurately done only by taking your weight while immersed in water). Most of us know what our "ideal" weight is based on what we feel comfortable and healthy weighing, but consult a physician if uncertain.

Table A-1 gives recommended amounts of food intake depending on what you have determined to be your ideal weight range. If your present weight is much above or below the ideal, this amount of food ought to bring you toward that goal. How much you lose or gain each week will depend on how far you have to go to reach that ideal.

Table A-1
Recommended Food Intake According to Ideal Body Weight

Women		Men	
Ideal Weight	Food Units*	Ideal Weight	Food Units
88-96	33-34	119-127	51-52
97-102	35-36	128-132	53-54
103-107	37-38	133-137	55-56
108-112	39-40	138-142	57-59
113-117	41-42	143-147	60-61
118-122	43-44	148-152	62-63
123-127	45-46	153-157	64-66
128-132	47-48	158-162	67-68
133-137	49-50	163-167	69-70
138-143	50-51	168-172	71-72
144-147	52-53	173-177	73-74
148-152	54-55	178-186	75-77
153-157	56-57	187-192	78-79
158-163	58-59	193-200	80-83

*Approximately 50 calories (kilocalories) each; see text.

Difference between sexes necessitated because of differing proportions of body fat.

Recommendations are for moderately active 30-50 years-olds. Add two units if under 30, and subtract two units if over 50. Add one to four units if very active, and subtract one to four units if underactive.

A Note about Food Units

In other publications, most listings of the nutritional value of food are based on nutrients provided per "serving." In this manner, dealing with a set "serving," a glass of cow's milk would contain more calcium than a sprig of broccoli. However, a glass of milk contains many more calories, mostly in the form of fat than the broccoli; one could get more calcium from broccoli in fewer calories than from milk. Thus, in these tables, the nutritive values of foods are given in terms of Equal Caloric Servings; the Food Units referred to are approximately 50 calories (kilocalories) each.

What Food to Choose

Choose the number of units recommended for your ideal weight by Table A-1 (of course, more than one unit of any food can be selected) and then verify that your total is close to 100% of each nutrient for the day. Table A-2 lists many foods produced in the United States, the amount of food that provides 50 Calories (one Food Unit), and the relative concentrations of five important nutrients in that food. The nutrient concentrations are listed as percentages of the U.S. Recommended Dietary Allowances (1980), and are intended as guidelines only.

Table A-2
Isocaloric (per 50 Calorie Food Unit) and Percentage of Adult U.S. Recommended Daily Allowance for Selected Nutrients

	Unit	Prot.	Iron	Cal.	Vit. A	Vit. C
Almonds	1 T	3	2	2	0	0
Apple	1 med (4 oz)	0	2	1	0	3
Apricots	3 med (3 oz)	2	3	2	29	17
Artichokes	1 med	6	7	7	2	16
Avocado	2 oz (about 1/7)	1	1	1	1	6
Barley	1.5 C, cooked	3	1	1	0	0
Beets	1 C, diced	4	5	3	0	17
Beet Greens	2 C	11	31	46	148	73
Black Beans	1/7 C, cooked	6	6	2	0	0
Black-eyed Peas	1/4 C, cooked	5	4	1	0	0
Blackberries	1/2 C	2	4	3	1	25
Bluberries	1/2 C	1	4	2	1	17
•Broccoli	1 stalk (1.25 C)	11	8	20	45	270
•Brussel Sprouts	1 C	13	9	6	8	225
•Cabbage	1.5 C, shredded	5	5	12	0	167
Cantalope	1/2 med, 5" dia.	2	4	3	60	105
Carrots	2 med, 6"	2	4	5	121	15
Cashews	1 T	3	2	0	0	0
•Cauliflower	2 C	11	8	6	1	220
Celery	3 C	5	5	15	7	45

	Unit	Prot.	Iron	Cal.	Vit. A	Vit. C
Cherries	1/2 C	2	2	2	8	10
Collard Greens	1 C	7	6	36	103	145
Corn	1 sm. ear, 4"	4	2	0	3	8
Cucumber	1 large, 10"	3	6	6	0	63
Dates	1 oz	1	3	1	0	0
Eggplant	1.25 C	4	7	3	0	12
Garbanzo Beans	1/7 C, cooked	5	6	3	0	0
Grapefruit (pink)	1/2 med	2	3	2	5	73
Grapes	1/2 C	1	2	1	1	5
Green Beans	1 2/3 C	5	8	12	10	40
Kale	1 2/3 C	11	11	25	120	167
Lentils	1/4 C, cooked	7	6	1	0	0
Lettuce (leaf)	10 leaves	9	19	21	48	75
Lima Beans	1/4 C	6	6	2	1	12
Maple Syrup	1 T	0	1	2	0	0
Molasses, b-strap	1 T	0	18	17	0	0
Mushrooms	1 1/4 C	11	8	2	0	8
Mustard Greens	1.5 C	8	21	35	120	167
Navy Beans	1/4 C, cooked	6	7	3	0	0
Nectarines	1/2 med (1.5" dia)	1	2	0	12	15
Oatmeal	1/2 C	4	4	1	0	0
Okra	16 pods (3")	7	4	19	8	57
Onion	1 med (3")	4	3	5	1	25
Orange	1 small (2.25")	1	2	6	2	95
Parsnips	1/2 C	2	2	4	0	13
Peach	1 large (3")	2	3	2	15	15
Peanuts	1 T	4	1	1	0	0
Peanut Butter	1/2 T	4	1	1	0	0
Pear	1/2 med	1	1	1	0	5
Peas	1/2 C	8	8	2	4	27
Pecans	1 T	1	1	1	0	0
Pepper, Green	3 med (11 oz)	5	8	3	9	467
Pepper, Red	2 med	4	4	2	66	500
Pineapple	2/3 C (1/4 lb)	1	3	2	1	26
Pinto Beans	1/7 C, cooked	6	5	2	0	0

The Most Noble Diet

	Unit	Prot.	Iron	Cal.	Vit. A	Vit. C
Plums	2 med	1	3	2	3	10
Popcorn (air pop)	2 C	3	2	0	0	0
Potato, White	3 oz (1/2 med)	3	2	1	0	17
Potato, Sweet	1/3 med	1	2	2	30	13
Prunes	3 med	1	4	1	3	1
Pumpkin Seeds	1 T (w/o shells)	5	6	4	0	0
Raisins	1 3/4 T	1	3	2	0	0
Raspberries	2/3 C	1	5	2	1	33
Rice, Brown	1/5 C, cooked	2	1	1	0	0
Rye, Whole	1/5 C, cooked (or 2 T flour)	3	3	1	0	0
Sesame Seeds	1 T	3	6	13	0	0
Sorghum Syrup	1 T	0	14	4	0	0
Soy Beans	1/5 c, cooked	7	5	3	0	0
Spinach	6 oz weight	9	22	21	140	83
Sprouts (bean)	1 1/4 C	9	9	3	0	41
Squash, Summer	1 1/2 C	5	7	9	12	50
Squash, Winter	1/3 C	2	3	2	30	15
Strawberries	1 C	2	8	4	1	146
Sunflower Seeds	1 T	4	3	1	0	0
Tangarine	1 large	1	2	5	4	50
Tofu (Bean Curd)	2 1/2 oz	11	8	12	0	0
Tomato	1 large	4	6	4	17	67
Turnip Greens	1 2/3 C	8	12	47	120	170
•Turnip Root	1 1/2 C	3	5	10	0	83
Walnuts	1 T	3	3	0	0	0
•Watercress	8 oz weight	9	28	47	122	333
Watermelon	4" x 4" wedge	2	6	2	12	25
Wheat, Whole	2 T flour, or 1 slice bread	4	4	1	0	0
Yeast, Nutritional	2 T	11	16	3	0	0
Zucchini	1 C	6	5	9	8	83

C = cup; T = tablespoon.   • = Cabbage family (Cruciferous) Vegetables   Vitamin A as beta-carotene

Calculated from tables in: U.S. Department of Agriculture. *Nutritive Value of Foods, Home and Garden Bulletin No. 72. 1971.* Government Printing Office, Washington, D.C.

A Note about Nutrients Listed in Table A-2

Protein, calcium, and iron are listed in Table A-2 because they are the major nutrients of concern to those who doubt the adequacy of a vegan diet (a diet which does not contain any animal products, including poultry, fish, seafood, lard, gelatin, eggs, and dairy products: milk, butter, yogurt, cheese, whey, and casein).

Because foods containing high amounts of Vitamin A and those containing a great deal of Vitamin C have been found to be protective against certain types of cancer, those nutrients are included in Table A-2 to facilitate planning a menu such that you receive enough of these nutrients. Vitamins A and C, in the form that it exists in the above foods, is not toxic in excess. Receiving more than 100% of the RDA of these nutrients from foods is not harmful, and may be helpful in preventing certain cancers. For protein and calcium, there is no advantage (and the possibility of toxicity) if consumption is habitually excessive (over 200% of RDA).

Vegetables from the cabbage family (cruciferous) also seem to have cancer-inhibiting properties, and these are marked in Table A-2 by an "•" so that they can included regularly.

It is important to note that with all of these nutrients, "cheating" (see Chapter 3) by taking pill supplements will not atone for an unbalanced diet. As far as cancer-prevention is concerned, there is no evidence that the benefits of eating foods containing protective substances can be duplicated by taking those substances in isolation.

A Sample Menu

Table A-3 shows a sample menu, calculated for a female with an ideal weight of 112 lbs., between the ages of 30 and 50. From Table A-1, her recommended food intake would be 40 Food Units (2000 Calories). As you will discover, it will not be necessary to painstakingly count your nutrient intake every day. With a whole-foods diet, any balance of fruits, vegetables (leafy and root), and seeds (grains, nuts, beans) will generally be more than adequate. For example, if your desirable intake is 50 food units a day, you have to eat only foods with a content of 2% per unit for each nutrient. Thus, any unit that has a score of 4 or more in one nutrient will allow you to have another unit with a score of zero for that nutrient.

Table A-3   A Sample Day's Menu Calculation

	# Units	Prot.	Iron	Cal.	Vit. A	Vit. C
Breakfast						
Blackberries, 1C	2	4	8	6	2	50
Plums, 2 med	1	2	6	4	6	20
WW bread, 2 slices	2	8	8	2	0	0
Morning Snack						
Strawberries, 1C	1	2	8	4	1	146
Cherries, 1C	2	4	4	4	16	20
Lunch						
Salad of:						
Lettuce, 5 leaves	0.5	4	9	10	24	37
Cabbage, 3/4C	0.5	2	2	6	0	83
Tomato, 1 large	1	4	6	4	17	67
Cucumber, 1/2 large	0.5	1	3	3	0	31
Sunflower Seeds, 3T	3	12	9	3	0	0
Nutritional Yeast, 1T	0.5	5	8	1	0	0
Carrot, 1 med	0.5	1	2	2	60	70
Walnuts, 2T	2	6	6	0	0	0
Afternoon Snack						
Watermellon, 4"x4"	1	2	6	2	12	25
Dinner						
Lima Beans, 1/2C	2	12	12	4	2	24
Corn, 2 med ears	3	12	6	0	6	24
Mustard Greens, 1 1/2C	1	8	21	35	120	167
Mushrooms, 1/2C	0.5	5	4	1	0	4
WW Bread, 2 slices	2	8	8	2	0	0
Peanut Buter, 3T	6	24	6	6	0	0
Grapes, 1C	2	2	4	2	2	10
Late-Night Snack						
Nectarines, 2 med	4	4	8	0	48	60
Pecans, 2T	2	2	2	2	0	0
Totals	40	134	156	103	316	838

Vegan Nutrition Basics

The meat, egg, and dairy lobbies – some of the largest and most taxpayer-subsidized industries – have disseminated false information about the human body's alleged need for animal products. Some of their falsehoods were based on skewed scientific studies, most of which were funded by the industries themselves. Even today, people insist humans must consume animal products, despite all the healthy people who don't!

Food is composed of carbohydrate, protein, fat, vitamins, minerals, and water. Carbohydrates, protein, and fat are known as energy nutrients because they supply calories.

Carbohydrates. These are the body's ideal energy source, and they also supply dietary fiber. One type of carbohydrate is the complex carbohydrate known as starch. Contrary to popular belief, starch is not fattening. In fact, starch is the nutrient we need in the greatest quantity: 70–80% of our daily calories should come from starchy foods. Complex carbohydrates are found only in plant foods – grains, legumes, vegetables, and fruits – thus, these foods should be the center of each meal.

Protein. The myth of protein as the best energy source was refuted decades ago. But old myths die hard, especially in this culture where protein is considered king. Many people believe that if they don't eat animal flesh, they will waste away. The body's need for protein is quite small, and excess protein consumption is linked to osteoporosis and other diseases. The average American consumes more than twice the recommended amount of protein. Only 10–15% of daily calories should come from protein. Foods from animals greatly exceed this amount. Protein needs are easily met on a plant-based diet as long as you consume enough calories and eat a variety of plant foods. Protein is not unique to meat, dairy products, and eggs: it is found in all whole foods: broccoli, wheat, lentils, rice, oatmeal, etc. Corn and carrots, potatoes and pasta – all contain protein.

Protein is used by the body for growth, maintenance, and repair after it has been broken down by the body's digestive system into its constituent amino acids. It is not true that some amino acids can be provided only by animal products. Nor is it true that vegetarians need to be careful about what

The Most Noble Diet

food combinations they make in order to get the right amounts of amino acids. If this were so, we and many of our friends would have wasted away long ago!

The human body utilizes 22 amino acids to form all the protein it needs. It can make all but eight of these on its own. These eight are obtained through one's diet. The concept of vegetable protein being incomplete is a myth. All grains, legumes, vegetables, nuts and seeds contain all the essential amino acids; only the proportions vary. The body absorbs the amino acids from plant protein slowly, and then keeps them in circulation for hours, so you don't have to eat large doses of all the essential amino acids in one sitting. Eating various foods throughout the day will supply your protein needs more than adequately.

Fat. In general, animal products are much higher in fat (especially saturated fat) than plant products. Every gram of fat contains 9 calories, whereas a gram of carbohydrate or protein contains 4 calories. Saturated fats are solid at room temperature and unsaturated fats are liquid. Hydrogenated oils – even vegetable oils – act like saturated fats. Beware: hydrogenated oils are found in many commercial baked goods and other processed foods. Cholesterol is a type of fat found only in animal products. (The human body makes its own required cholesterol. It needs no dietary sources.) Saturated fat intake has been linked to atherosclerosis, the buildup of cholesterol and fat in the artery walls, and other diseases. Only three plant sources are high in saturated fats: coconuts, palm oil, and chocolate. Almost all animal products have high percentages of saturated fats. Animal products contain no fiber, but do have cholesterol. Almost all plant products have fiber and none have any significant cholesterol content. Red meat derives 50–70% of its calories from fat; chicken, even with the skin removed, is 30–40% fat. The typical American consumes 40–50% of calories from fat.

The easiest way to reduce your fat consumption is to reduce your intake of animal products. While others recommend an "achievable" amount (up to 30%!), for optimal health it is recommended that fat supply no more than 10–15% of daily calories.

Calcium. Although milk has large amounts of calcium, its calcium is not as available to your body as the calcium in most leafy green vegetables, broccoli, tofu, corn tortillas, legumes, and figs. This is because of the high level of phosphorus in milk, as well as excess protein. Phosphorus and excess protein (which is comprised of amino acids) make your blood acidic, and the calcium in milk (or your bones) is used as calcium carbonate, a base, to stabilize the acid level in your blood. A vegan thus does not need to eat as much calcium as someone who eats dairy products. A balanced vegan diet will provide you with adequate amounts of calcium.

Osteoporosis, the loss of calcium from the bones, is much more prevalent in meat-eaters and has been linked to excessive protein intake. Because animal flesh is much higher in protein than vegetable-based foods, meat-eaters (including those who eat fish, which is extremely high in protein) are more likely to have excessive protein intake and so have osteoporosis more often than vegans.

Iron. The following foods contain significant amounts of iron: molasses, sorghum, dark leafy green vegetables, beet greens, whole and enriched grains, legumes, potatoes, artichokes, beans, grains, and many fruits. Include a good source of Vitamin C to help the body absorb iron more efficiently. Good sources of Vitamin C are citrus fruits and juices, strawberries, green peppers, melons, potatoes, and broccoli.

Vitamin B-12. Only trace amounts of Vitamin B-12 are necessary, and it is stored in your body for months. B-12 is made by bacteria, and is found (besides in animal products) on the surface of raw organic vegetables, in nutritional (not brewers) yeast (available at health food stores), and in some fortified cereals (Grape nuts, Total, Nutrigrain, and others). Some soy products are fortified with B-12. It is prudent to eat something with B-12 occasionally.

The Most Noble Diet

APPENDIX B
NO BANANAS? WHAT ABOUT POTASSIUM?

The recommendation that we curtail our consumption of bananas (Chapter 7) may cause some alarm on the part of those concerned about their potassium intake. Potassium is an essential mineral that, among other things, helps to regulate blood pressure, especially when a body is overloaded with sodium (from salt, etc.). Some diuretic medications, usually given to reduce blood pressure in those with hypertension, actually flush the potassium out of the body, creating a potentially deficient situation.

Well-meaning physicians, nurses, and even some dietitians advise anyone concerned to eat a banana every day. This is probably done because bananas are a reasonably good source of potassium, are generally well liked (because of their sweetness), and are typically quite inexpensive (for less than ethical reasons, as previously discussed).

Table B-1
Potassium (mg) per 100 Cal

Mushrooms	1450
Tomatoes	950
Broccoli	950
Green Beans	590
Potatoes	560
Lima Beans	520
Strawberries	480
Peaches	480
Oranges	440
Bananas	440

Source: *USDA Agricultural Handbook*, No. 456

However, the general public has taken this advice to mean that bananas have a monopoly on potassium, or are at least the best source of it. The truth is that, on a calorie-for-calorie basis, other fruits and many vegetables have a much higher potassium content than bananas (Table B-1).

The sweetness of bananas is a clue to their high calorie content. A typical banana contains 100 Calories, while most other fruits and vegetables have a much lower calorie content compared to their size. The potassium in a 100 Calorie banana can be found in one tomato (45 Calories) or 3/4 cup cooked mushrooms (30 Calories). In this nation of over-eaters, health professionals ought not recommend the higher caloric choices for obtaining our nutrients.

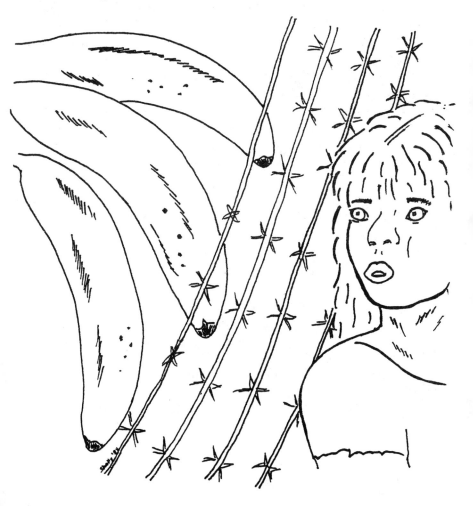

The Most Noble Diet

APPENDIX C
A NOTE ABOUT FOOD COMBINING

There is much controversy over whether it is important to eat certain foods together or separately. There are two concepts involved in these food combining discussions.

Food Separation

The first, more accurately described as "food separating," has been expounded by advocates of the Natural Hygiene[38] approach to diet. This school of thought is nearly a century old, but was brought to popular attention by Harvey and Marilyn Diamond in their 1980s best-seller *Fit for Life*. Various rules for not mixing certain fruits with certain vegetables, starchy foods with high-protein foods, etc. are central facets of this dietary regime. The theory behind this is that requiring the digestive system to produce a great variety of enzymes leads to less-than-efficient food absorption because incomplete digestion occurs.

Although many overweight people might welcome "incomplete" digestion as a way to stuff themselves without bulging further the next day, the scientific challenge to the theory is that all natural, whole foods are a combination of different proteins, fats, starches, and sugars. To handle this, the human digestive system is capable of producing thousands of different enzymes at once, even for foods never before eaten. If this were not so, everyone would have serious stomach pains every time they ate a mixed meal, and certainly every time they ate something new.

Natural hygienists counter that the mixtures of nutrients that occur in any one food are "natural" mixtures, and thus are more easily handled by the body. This idea has merit from a common-sense standpoint, and is quite possibly a key

---

[38] Natural Hygiene is more than simply an approach to diet, but an entire way of looking at the human body, starting with the idea that all healing must be initiated by the body itself.

component in the success of Natural Hygiene in treating people suffering from less-than-optimal health. When ill, the body is busy using its protein to build antibodies to fight disease. Since enzymes are built from protein as well, it makes sense that production of these substances will be less than optimal at these times. Even many healthy people have a food or combination of foods that does not "agree" with them.

Food Combining

The second concept – "food combining" – comes from the orthodox medical/nutritional community. Much has been made (mostly by those denigrating a vegetarian diet) of the "necessity" of combining amino acids for proper protein construction. It is of course true that an individual on a minimalist diet can get more use from two "incomplete" proteins if eaten together. However, most of us eat much more protein than we need anyway, and because all plant proteins are complete if eaten in adequate quantities, it is not necessary to purposely seek out combinations (although this doesn't hurt as long as it is not used as an excuse to overeat)

Another issue is synergism of nutrients, where one food boosts usage of another. Frequently cited as an example is that Vitamin C enhances the body's absorption of iron, so that if you eat two foods together, each rich in one nutrient, you are able to utilize more of the iron than if you ate them at separate meals. Grains are a good source of iron, but contain almost no Vitamin C; the saying "One cannot live by bread alone" may have been an observation of the anemia (or scurvy) that resulted when there were no fruits or fresh vegetables around to eat with the bread. Dark green leafy vegetables are excellent sources of both iron and Vitamin C (though the latter only if not overcooked), so both nutrients can be obtained without violating a Natural Hygienist's avoidance of food combining.

APPENDIX D
THE QUESTION OF HONEY

Bees ingest nectar from flowers and then regurgitate it as honey, making it, technically, an animal-derived product. During the honey collection process, many of bees can be killed and mutilated. Although there is no scientific consensus on whether bees (or other insects) can suffer as vertebrate animals do, this killing is unnecessary, given the chance that the bees do suffer.

Honey is in no way an essential food for human beings. As a sweetener it holds no advantages over purely plant-derived syrups such as molasses, maple syrup, sorghum, barley malt, etc. In fact, most of the alternatives contain more nutrients (molasses much more); it is only in comparison with highly-refined sweeteners like white sugar and corn syrup that honey seems superior.

In addition, honey causes a more severe jump in blood glucose than other sweeteners, since it contains much free glucose that is immediately absorbed into the blood. Honey has also been implicated as a cause of infant botulism[39] and is thus not medically recommended for babies under six months.

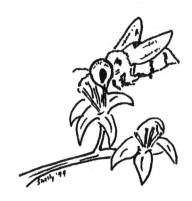

---

[39] Most food poisoning comes from animal-derived products.

APPENDIX E
NOBLE RECIPES

Following are some recipes for an ethical and healthy life – for you, the earth, the animals, and other people. Leaf through and see the variety there is to eat. It should be clear that following an ethical vegan diet does not mean living in a culinary wasteland. Rather, it allows us to become aware of the great diversity of foods available. More importantly, being a moral, compassionate person is the greatest accomplishment an individual can achieve.

With some simple planning, eating well does not need to be a hassle. Here are some tips: Plan a weekly menu ahead of time and prepare a shopping list so you can get everything in one trip to the store(s), with side trips later to purchase fresh vegetables. Get in the habit of soaking beans overnight. Go to a farmer's market for a wide variety and good prices on fruits and vegetables. Make extra at dinner and have the leftovers for lunch during the week.

These recipes are merely our versions – take notes, create your own. Vary a recipe, add or substitute vegetables, nuts or seeds, or spices. Serve a French dish with a Thai one. Why not?

For quicker meals, most natural foods stores have boxed (or better yet, in bulk) vegan foods: tabouli, hummus, instant refried beans, soup mixes, grain "burger" mixes , etc. Canned soups, beans, and pasta sauces are also available. Look for new vegan items, which are constantly appearing on the market. (Some may be available in your area grocery store.) White Wave makes soy-based vegan "yogurt." Tofutti, and Living Lightly make low-fat or non-fat versions of non-dairy desserts.

Travel Ideas. Stock a small cooler with fruit, raw vegetables (like carrots), tomato or other juices, bean dip, hummus, or peanut butter (but watch the fat). Take pretzels (whole grain, if possible), cereals, popcorn, fat-free cookies, crackers, bagels, rice cakes, tortilla chips (Guiltless Gourmet makes baked tortilla chips that are very low fat). This can make traveling less expensive and more pleasant.

Sweeteners. Many vegans use fructose or turbinado sugar for the dry sugars; maple syrup, molasses, or Fruitsource as liquid. Sugar is sugar – there are minerals in molasses, but otherwise simple sugars don't provide any vitamins or minerals. Try not to overdo the sugar, whichever you decide to use. Only low-fat dessert recipes are listed here. You'll find plenty of high-fat recipes in other cookbooks!

Spices. All entrees are *conservatively* spiced. Spicier folks might like to double the onions, triple the spices, and quadruple the garlic.

Servings. All are approximate and depend on whether the dish is to be an entree or a side dish. Except those with peanut butter or a lot of tofu (lower fat tofu is now available, and all tofu is relatively low in saturated fat), all recipes are low fat. Use water to sauté veggies to reduce fat content further. Enjoy!

Guidelines for Making Any Recipe More Noble
• Use organically grown items whenever possible.
• Substitute locally grown items for imported food, such as ripe pears or even squash for bananas.
• Steam or bake when cooking foods to avoid having to use fats for frying.
• Use whole fruits or squeeze your own juice, and utilize the pulp in some way. Most commercial juice plants sell their pulp for animal feed at a very low price. This helps keep the price of animal flesh sold for consumption lower than it should be.

Some Other Helpful Recipe Books:
The Cookbook for People who Love Animals, Umatilla, FL: Gentle World, 1987.

The McDougall Plan and the *McDougall Plan Recipes, Vols. 1 & II*, New Century Publishers, Piscataway, NJ, 1983, 1985, and 1986, respectively.

Soul Vegetarian Cookbook, Communications Press, (P.O. Box 26063, Washington, DC 20001), 1992.

Wasserman, Debra, *Simply Vegan: Quick Vegetarian Meals*, The Vegetarian Resource Group (P.O. Box 1463, Baltimore MD 21203), 1991.

SALAD DRESSINGS

Garlicky Caesar Dressing

4–5 cloves fresh garlic
1 t olive oil
1 t red wine vinegar
2 t balsamic vinegar
juice of one lemon
1–2 drops hot pepper sauce

With a fork, mash garlic in olive oil, then whisk in remaining ingredients. Let dressing sit overnight in refrigerator for stronger garlic flavor. Serve over a green salad of your choice.

Super Salad dressing

2 whole tomatoes or 6 oz. tomato or V-8 juice,
celery stalks, carrot strips, bell pepper pieces
raw onion and/or garlic to taste
2 T lemon juice and/or vinegar
spices and seasonings to taste

Blend all ingredients in blender, adding more hard vegetables (celery, carrots) to obtain desired thickness.
This can also be used as a sauce for baked potatoes or steamed vegetables, or as a dip for raw vegetables.

Balsamic Vinaigrette

1/3 C balsamic vinegar
1/4 C apple cider vinegar
1/4 C water
1 T Dijon mustard
1 T minced fresh garlic
1 T minced fresh parsley
1 t apple juice concentrate

Whisk together all ingredients in a small bowl. Enjoy over a vegetable salad of your choice. Serves 3-4.

The Most Noble Diet

Zero-Fat Herb Dressing

1/4 C tomato or V-8 juice (6 oz can)
1/4 C red-wine vinegar
1 T minced fresh parsley
1 T chopped chives or scallions
1 clove garlic, crushed
1/2 t salt
pinch dried savory or oregano
pinch sugar
pinch cayenne pepper
freshly ground black pepper

Combine with a blender. Enjoy over green salad. Serves 3-4.

SALADS

Marinated Broccoli and/or Cauliflower

1C vinegar
1 t dill
2 T each: chopped onion, parsley, celery
1 t mustard

Blend above in blender on medium speed for 10 seconds.
　　Pour over:
　　2 heads cauliflower or broccoli, or one of each, raw or lightly
steamed, broken into bite-sized pieces.
　　Refrigerate for 2 hours before serving.

Yam Yai (Thai Salad)

Salad
1 head lettuce (preferably butter lettuce), torn into bite-sized pieces
1/2 cucumber, sliced
1 carrot, sliced or slivered
Orange slices (garnish)
2 T chopped fresh cilantro (garnish)
2 T chopped unsalted dry-roasted peanuts (garnish)

Dressing
1/4 C natural peanut butter
4 T water
1 T fresh minced ginger root
1 T soy sauce
4 T lime juice (or less to taste)
1 t sugar (or more to taste)
1 clove garlic, minced
Dash hot chili paste

Arrange lettuce on large platter. Top with cucumbers and carrots, and garnish with orange and cilantro. In a bowl, mix together all dressing ingredients and pour on top of vegetables. Sprinkle with chopped peanuts if desired. Good with Pad Thai, or Spring Rolls.

Fat-Free Coleslaw

Dressing
1/3 C cider vinegar
2 T Dijon mustard
1 T low-sodium soy sauce
2 t turbinado or other sugar
1/2 t celery seed (optional)
1/2 t caraway seed
1/4 t ground black pepper

Salad
2 C shredded green cabbage
2 C shredded red cabbage
1 carrot, julienned (or chopped)
1 red bell pepper, julienned
1 green bell pepper, julienned
1 yellow bell pepper, julienned
1/4 C finely chopped scallions
1/4 C minced fresh parsley

Mix dressing ingredients together in small jar. Combine salad vegetables in a large bowl. Pour dressing over vegetables and toss to coat. Refrigerate at least 1 hour to blend flavors. Serves 4-6.

Hot Potato Salad

6 – 8 medium potatoes (any kind)
1 medium chopped onion (optional)
1/2 C chopped cabbage (and/or green beans)
1/3 C peas
2 T minced dill pickle
1 diced red or green bell pepper
1/4 C water
1/2 C apple cider vinegar
1 t fructose or other sweetener
2 T prepared mustard
Salt and pepper to taste

Boil whole unpeeled potatoes for 20 minutes, or until tender when pierced with fork. Drain well and allow to cool slightly. Cut into bite-sized pieces and transfer to a large bowl. Add onion, pickle. Steam other veggies for a few minutes and add to potatoes. Toss.

In a small saucepan, combine water, vinegar, sweetener, and mustard. Bring to a boil. Simmer 2 min., then pour over potatoes. Toss well, adjust seasonings and serve at once. Serves 4-6. Also good cold.

Sweet and Spicy Couscous Salad

1/2 C raisins
1/4 C orange juice
1/4 C lemon juice
1/4 t ground cinnamon
1/2 t salt
1/8 t cayenne pepper (or more to taste)

3 C water
1 1/2 C couscous, preferably whole wheat
1 medium carrot, finely chopped
1 C green or yellow wax beans (cut into 1/4 inch pieces)
1 medium red or green bell pepper, seeded and finely   chopped
1/2 C peas
1/4 C finely chopped fresh mint or parsley

Put the raisins, orange juice, lemon juice, cinnamon, salt, and cayenne in a jar. Cover with lid and shake until ingredients are well mixed.

In a medium saucepan, bring the water to a boil. Stir in couscous. Immediately remove from heat, cover, and let stand until the water is absorbed, about 6 min. Transfer the couscous to a large bowl, and fluff with a fork. Cool.

Steam the carrot, beans, peas, and bell pepper in a steamer basket, covered, about 3 min. They should still crunch. Rinse under cold water, drain, and cool.

Stir the steamed vegetables and mint or parsley into the couscous. Shake the dressing and pour it over the salad. Stir until well coated. Refrigerate for at least 30 min. to allow flavors to blend. Serves 4-6.

The Most Noble Diet

Spicy Black Bean and Lentil Salad

2 C cooked black beans
2 C cooked red lentils
1 t dry mustard
3 T minced fresh garlic
1 T fresh parsley
1 T minced fresh cilantro
1/2 C rice or other vinegar
3 T lemon juice
1 t salt (or to taste)
2 – 3 T olive oil (optional)
1 t crushed red pepper
1 small head leaf lettuce, washed and torn
2 large red bell peppers, cut into 8 rings each
2 large red potatoes, cooked and thinly sliced
1/2 cup grated carrots or raw beets

Place black beans in one bowl, lentils in another. In a third bowl, whisk together mustard, garlic, parsley, cilantro, vinegar, lemon juice, salt, oil, and red pepper. Divide mixture equally between beans and lentils; cover and let marinate for 1 hour in the refrigerator.

Line 6 salad plates with lettuce leaves, then top with rings of red pepper. Arrange small piles of potatoes, carrots or beets, beans, and lentils on each plate, then drizzle remaining marinade over all. Serve immediately.

Cold Marinated Vegetables

6 carrots, grated
1 C green beans, steamed
1 C shredded cabbage
1 cucumber, coarsely grated
1 C bean sprouts
2 cloves garlic, minced
1/2 – 2 t crushed red pepper
3 T turbinado or other sugar
3 T rice or cider vinegar
1 T lime or lemon juice
1 – 2 t turmeric (optional)

Place vegetables in a large bowl. Mix together garlic, crushed red pepper, sugar, vinegar, lime or lemon juice, and turmeric if desired (gives yellow color). Pour mixture over vegetables. Toss thoroughly, cover and chill for at least 4 hours. Serve cold or at room temperature. Makes 4 servings.

Thai Noodle Salad

4 oz. dried thin rice noodles
2 carrots, shredded
1/2 medium cabbage, finely chopped
4 cloves garlic, minced
1 T minced fresh ginger root
3 green onions, chopped
1/2 – 1 t toasted sesame oil
1 – 2 T turbinado or other sugar
Juice of 1 lime
2 T low-sodium soy sauce
2 t chili powder
1 T tomato paste
2 t chopped peanuts (optional)
2 T chopped fresh basil, mint, or cilantro leaves (optional)

Place rice noodles in a heat-proof bowl. Pour boiling water over them to cover completely. Let noodles soak for 7 minutes, then drain thoroughly.

Grate carrots and finely shred cabbage into a large bowl. Set aside.

In a large, heavy saucepan, sauté garlic, ginger, and green onions in sesame oil, tossing frequently, for about 2 minutes. Whisk in sugar, lime juice, soy sauce, chili powder, and tomato paste. Bring to a boil, then reduce heat and simmer for about 4 minutes. Remove from heat and let cool to room temperature.

Add noodles and sauce to carrot-cabbage mixture. Toss well and place on a serving platter. If desired, garnish with peanuts and basil, mint or cilantro leaves. Serves 4.

The Most Noble Diet

AMERICAN

Oat Burgers

2 C rolled oats
2 C water
2 T tamari (soy sauce)
1 small onion, chopped
1/2 t crushed garlic or garlic powder
2 T sunflower seeds or chopped walnuts
2 T sesame seeds.

Combine first three in sauce pan and bring to a boil. Reduce heat and simmer 5 minutes. Let stand until cool.

Add remaining ingredients. Form into patties, place on non-stick cookie sheet, and bake at 325° for 35 minutes. Turn them over after the first 20 minutes.

Twice-Baked Potatoes

2 large Idaho potatoes
1/2 C water
1 medium onion, chopped
1/2 t cumin
1/4 t curry powder (or more to taste)
1 1/2 T nutritional yeast
2 T soy sauce
paprika

Bake potatoes at 400° for about 1 hour. (Make sure to pierce them in a few places with a fork before baking. Also, these keep well in the fridge, and are good for lunches. Make a double or triple batch while you have the oven on.)

Sauté onions in a little water, add cumin, curry and yeast. Stir in remaining water, and soy sauce. Bring to a boil to dissolve all seasonings. Set aside.

Cool potatoes slightly. Roll on a counter with the palm of your hand to loosen pulp. Cut lengthwise and scoop out pulp into a mixing bowl. Try not to break skins.

Add onion mixture to potato pulp. Mix with a hand blender. Spoon filling into potato skins and sprinkle with paprika. Broil for 5 minutes. Serves 2 as written.

Tofu w/Key West Barbecue Sauce

1 lb extra-firm tofu
2 T unbleached white flour
2 T yellow cornmeal
2 t nutritional yeast
1/2 t salt (optional)
1/4 freshly ground black pepper
2 T prepared yellow mustard
4 T oil

Sauce
1/2 C tomato sauce
1/3 C turbinado or other sugar
2 T lime juice
2 cloves garlic, finely minced
1 small onion, finely minced
4 T vegetarian Worcestershire sauce
1 t hot pepper sauce

Cut tofu on short end into 1/4 inch slices. Drain on a towel or paper towels for about 30 min.

On a plate, mix flour, cornmeal, nutritional yeast, salt, and pepper. Brush drained tofu on both sides with mustard, then roll in cornmeal mixture.

Heat 1 tablespoon oil in a heavy skillet over medium heat; carefully place 4 slices of tofu in skillet, without crowding, and sauté until golden brown. Drain on paper towels. Keep warm in a low oven while cooking remaining tofu in remaining oil.

In a heavy medium-sized saucepan, combine all sauce ingredients. Bring to a boil, reduce heat, and simmer on low heat for 20 – 30 min. Pour sauce over tofu. Serve with a grain and a green salad. Serves 4-6.

Cheezy Sauce

2 C water
4 T cornstarch or arrowroot powder
1T flour
4 – 5 T prepared mustard (any style)
1/2 C nutritional yeast

Combine with a mixer or blender. Cook over medium heat, stirring, until thick. Serve over pasta, rice, potatoes, veggies. Use as a dip for pretzels, breadsticks, etc. This is the best non-cheese sauce we've ever tasted.

Mexican variation:
instead of mustard, add
1/4 C salsa
2 T lemon juice
1/2 t onion powder

Cook as above. (All other ingredients the same.) Serve as a dip with tortilla chips, bake on burritos, etc. Sauce thickens as it cools.

TJ's Famous Sloppy Joes
(thanks to Tom Rudnick)

3/4 C dry lentils
1/4 C brown rice
1 t oil
1/4 t black pepper
1/2 t cumin
1/4 t salt

1 small carrot, sliced
1 med. onion, diced
1 med. green pepper, diced
1 med. tomato, chopped
2 cloves garlic

2 C texturized vegetable protein
1/4 C red wine
1 1/2 T soy sauce
1 1/2 T vinegar
1/4 t paprika
1 t basil

2 t chili powder
2 t wet mustard
1/2 t sugar
12 oz tomato paste

In large saucepan, cook first set of ingredients in 3 cups of water for about 3/4 hour. In frying pan, sauté second set of ingredients in 1 T oil. Combine and let soak third set of ingredients. Combine first three sets with fourth. Heat. Serve on bread or buns. Also tasty on baked potatoes.

Neat Loaf

1 C cooked brown rice
1 C TVP soaked in 1 1/2 C water, or 1 C wheat germ
1 C quick oats
1 C finely chopped walnuts or sunflower seeds, or 1 C Grape Nuts cereal
1 C chopped mushrooms
1 onion finely chopped
1 med. bell pepper, finely chopped
1 med. carrot, finely chopped
1/2 t thyme
1/2 t marjoram
1/2 t sage
2 T soy sauce
2 T prepared mustard
4 oz tomato sauce

Combine ingredients and form into loaf. Bake at 350° for 60 min. in loaf pan. Make baked potatoes while you are at it. Serve with a green salad.

Potato-Apple Bake

2 large crisp, sweet apples
2 lbs red or white potatoes (about 5 – 6 cups sliced)
Salt and pepper
1 onion, chopped
Freshly grated nutmeg

Preheat oven to 350°. Core and thinly slice apples, and potatoes.
Lightly oil a 9x13 baking dish. Layer in half of the potatoes,
onions, apples. Sprinkle with spices. Repeat. Cover with foil or
baking sheet and bake 45 min. Serves 4.

Bubble and Squeak

10 – 12 medium potatoes, steamed until tender, and peeled
(works best when potatoes are steamed ahead of time and
chilled)
1 t olive oil
1 onion, chopped
1/2 medium cabbage, finely chopped (approx. 4 C)
4 T water
salt and pepper to taste

Grate potatoes. Sauté onion in olive oil (use a large wok– this
makes a large amount), add cabbage and water, continue
sautéing until cabbage is bright green and soft. Add potatoes
and salt and pepper to taste. Mix thoroughly and cook until
potatoes are heated through. Serves 4-6.

Vegetable-Laden Three-Bean Chili

1 green bell pepper
1 red bell pepper
1 yellow bell pepper
2 medium bulbs fennel
1 T virgin olive oil
1/4 t crushed red pepper
1 T cumin seeds
1 t dried oregano
2 T chili powder
3 med. tomatoes, peeled and chopped (16 oz. can diced tomatoes)
1 1/2 C cut green beans
1 3/4 C cooked kidney beans
1 3/4 C cooked black beans
1 3/4 C cooked white beans
Water or tomato juice as needed
Salt and freshly ground pepper to taste
1/2 C chopped cilantro or parsley

Seed bell peppers and cut into 1/2 inch squares. Remove tops from the fennel bulbs, cut out the core with a small knife and finely chop. Set aside.

Warm oil, crushed red pepper, coriander and cumin in a heavy 4-quart saucepan over moderate heat. Fry until seasonings darken slightly.

Add peppers, fennel, oregano, and chili powder, sauté for 5 min. Stir in tomatoes and all beans and bring to a boil. Reduce heat to low and simmer for 30 min., adding water or tomato juice as needed. Season with salt and pepper, stir in cilantro or parsley. Serves 6.

The Most Noble Diet

Black Bean Chili

2 C black beans
6 C water
1 bunch cilantro, chopped (optional)
1 T cumin seed
1 T oregano
1 t paprika
1/2 t cayenne
2 t olive oil
1 large onion, chopped
1 bell pepper, diced
2 cloves garlic, minced
1 1/2 C tomatoes, chopped
1/2 t salt
1/4 C chopped green onion for topping

Wash beans thoroughly and remove and debris. Place in a large kettle and add water and chopped cilantro. Cover loosely and simmer until tender, about 2 hours.

In a small dry skillet, heat the herbs, and toast them until fragrant.

In a larger skillet, sauté the onion for 2 – 3 min. Stir in the bell pepper, garlic, and herbs and sauté until the onion ins soft and golden. Add to the beans, along with tomatoes and salt. Simmer for 30 min. (the flavor improves upon longer cooking). Serve with chopped green onion.

Spicy Pumpkin Soup

2 onions, chopped
4 cloves garlic, minced
1/2 t mustard seed
1/2 t turmeric
1/2 t ginger
1/2 t cumin
1/4 t cinnamon
1/4 t salt
1/8 t cayenne
1 C water

1 T lemon juice
2 C cooked pumpkin (16 oz. can)
2 T maple syrup or other sugar
1 C soymilk (lite, if possible)

Sauté onion until soft and golden, then add garlic, spices, and salt. Cook 2 min. over low heat, stirring constantly, then whisk in water, lemon juice, pumpkin, sweetener, and soymilk. Remove from heat.

Puree soup with a hand blender until very smooth. Heat again until hot and steamy, about 10 min. Serves 4.

Crispy Crackers

2 C whole wheat pastry flour
2 t baking powder
1/2 t salt (optional)

1/2 C nutritional yeast OR
2 t caraway OR
1 t basil and 1 t oregano OR
1/2 t garlic powder and 1 t chili powder
OR your own combination of spices

2/3 – 1 C water

Mix dry ingredients. Add water until able to knead into a smooth ball. Roll out on a lightly oiled baking sheet and cut into shapes or score with a knife. Sprinkle more spices on top, if desired. Bake at 350° for 10 min. Good with spicy pumpkin or other soup.

The Most Noble Diet

Spicy Corn Bread

5 T olive oil (or water)
1 medium red bell pepper, seeded and finely chopped
1 fresh hot chili pepper, seeded and minced
1 C soymilk
2 T lemon juice
1 C whole wheat pastry flour
1 C yellow stone-ground cornmeal
1 t baking powder
1 t baking soda
1 t salt
kernels from one ear of sweet corn (or 3/4 C frozen corn, thawed)

Preheat oven to 350°. Lightly oil 8x8 baking pan with olive oil and dust with cornmeal, tapping out the excess.

Heat 1 tablespoon oil or water in a frying pan over medium heat. Add bell pepper and chili pepper and cook, stirring, for 5 min. Remove peppers from pan and cool completely.

Place soymilk, oil or water, and lemon juice in a small bowl and stir together.

Whisk the flour, cornmeal, baking powder, baking soda, and salt together in a large bowl until combined. Add soymilk mixture and combine, using as few strokes as possible so as to not overmix the batter. Fold in peppers and corn.

Spread the batter evenly in the prepared pan. Bake until a toothpick inserted into the center comes out clean, 20 – 25 min. Cool for 5 min. and cut into squares. Serve hot or cold. Good with chili.

SAUCES (for stir fry)

Peanut Sauce

1/2 C peanut butter or almond butter
2 T sesame oil
3 T soy sauce
3 T lemon juice
3 T liquid sweetener
1/2 t curry powder and/or coriander
1/4 C green onions
3 T fresh ground ginger
3 cloves garlic, minced

In small saucepan, heat oil and sauté onions, garlic, and ginger.
Reduce heat and add other ingredients, stirring constantly.
Serve over veggies and rice or noodles.

Ginger-Sesame Reduction Sauce

1/4 C water
1/4 C dry sherry or vegetable stock
1 T grated fresh ginger root
1/2 C minced green onions
2 cloves garlic
1 – 2 t dark sesame oil
1/4 C maple syrup or other sweetener
1/4 C low sodium tamari or soy sauce
2 t arrowroot

In a heavy saucepan, simmer water, sherry or stock, ginger
root, green onions, garlic, sesame oil and sweetener over
medium-high heat for 20 – 30 min., until sauce is reduced to
half its original volume.

In a small bowl, combine tamari or soy sauce with
arrowroot, stirring to remove lumps. Add slowly to reduced
sauce and cook, stirring constantly, until slightly thickened.
Adjust seasonings and serve.

Ginger Sauce

Clove of garlic, mashed
2 T grated ginger root
1 bell pepper, chopped
1 firm tomato, chopped
1 small onion, finely chopped
2 T catsup
2 T soy sauce
1 t sugar
1 C water or broth
1 t sesame oil
1 T cornstarch mixed with 3 T water

Heat oil in wok. When hot, add ginger & garlic and cook for 5 sec. to bring out flavor. Add all ingredients except cornstarch and cook for 5 min. at boiling. Thicken with cornstarch and serve over veggies and/or tofu, and rice or noodles.

ASIAN

Indonesian-Style Baked Tofu

1 1/2 t sesame oil
1 1/2 t pressed or minced garlic
1 1/2 t grated fresh ginger root
3/4 C mild vegetable stock or water
3 1/2 T peanut butter
1 T soy sauce
1 T lemon juice
1 1/2 t brown rice or other vinegar
pinch cayenne or more to taste
salt and pepper to taste
8 oz extra-firm tofu, drained

Combine all ingredients except tofu with a mixer or blender. Preheat oven to 325°

Cut tofu lengthwise into 1/4 to 3/8 inch slices and arrange in lightly oiled baking dish. Pour sauce over tofu, and bake for 30 min. Serve on brown rice, garnished with green onion or cilantro, if desired.

Spring Rolls

1 large onion, chopped
1 bunch green onions, chopped
1 T minced fresh ginger
2 C shredded carrots
4 C chopped or shredded cabbage
1 can water chestnuts, sliced
2 C bean sprouts
1/4 C soy sauce
1 t sesame oil
pepper
Chinese 5-spice powder

1 package phyllo dough

These are worth the time. Be patient. Make sure to thaw the phyllo in the fridge the night before, and at room temp for 2 hours before making spring rolls.

Heat wok, sauté onions, ginger, green onion in sesame oil. Add a little (2 T) water. Add carrots and cabbage, more water, if necessary. Cook for a few minutes, stirring, flipping. Add water chestnuts and bean sprouts, cook for a few more minutes. Add soy sauce, pepper and 5 spice to taste. Set aside to cool.

Preheat oven to 500°. Lay out phyllo onto a clean counter, cover with a damp cloth to prevent drying out. Remove sheet from the pile, fold in half to form a rectangle. . ALWAYS cover remaining phyllo immediately. You need to work quickly. Place about 1/4 C of filling towards one end. Fold the phyllo over the filling and roll twice. Fold the sides in and roll again. Place on lightly oil baking sheet. Cover with paper towel that has been lightly oiled with sesame oil until all rolls are prepared. Bake for 10-15 min. Makes about 16 (depending on how many sheets of phyllo you use.)

Serve with sweet and sour sauce, hot mustard, and/or soy sauce.

Curry-Laced Tomato-Lentil Broth

1 1/2 C lentils
4 C water

1 lb can crushed tomatoes
1 C water
1 1/2 t ground cumin
2 t ground coriander
1/4 – 1/2 cayenne
1 minced onion
2 cloves minced garlic
2 t salt
1 T lemon juice
1 t mustard seed

Cook lentils in 4 C water over medium heat for 25 min. Cover, reduce heat to simmer and cook for 10 min. more.
　　Add all other ingredients and cook for 10 min.

Hot and Spicy Noodles with Vegetables

1 t sesame or peanut oil
1/4 C rice wine (or white wine)
2 T grated fresh ginger root
2 cloves garlic, minced
1 C thinly sliced carrots
1 C broccoli florets
1 C thinly sliced green cabbage
2 green onions, diagonally sliced
1/4 C water
1/2 – 1 t cayenne pepper
1 T turbinado or other sugar
4 C cooked rice noodles (or rice)
Low sodium soy sauce to taste

In a wok over medium-high heat, heat oil and wine until bubbling. Add ginger, garlic, carrots and broccoli. Stir fry until carrots soften slightly, about 5 min. Add cabbage and green onions, cover and cook 3 min. With a slotted spoon, remove vegetables to platter and set aside.

Add water, cayenne and sugar to wok and heat until bubbling. Add noodles and stir fry until heated through. Add soy sauce to taste. Serves 4.

Pad Thai

Noodles and Sauce:
8 oz rice or 1 lb soba noodles (heartier)
1/2 C vinegar
1/3 C tomato paste
1/3 C water
1/4 C fructose or other sweetener
1 large onion, chopped
8 cloves garlic, minced
2 inch piece of fresh ginger, minced (optional)
2 green chilies, seeded and minced

Veggies:
1 can water chestnuts
2 C bean sprouts
2 C chopped carrots

Garnishes:
limes
chopped peanuts
sliced green onion

Prepare noodles, drain and set aside. Mix vinegar, tomato paste, water and sugar. Set aside. In a wok, stir fry onion, garlic and ginger in water (or a little sesame oil). Add carrots, water chestnuts and a little water and stir fry for a few minutes. Add vinegar mixture, bean sprouts, and noodles, stir and cook until sauce thickens (about 5 minutes). Serve with garnishes. Serves about 4.

FRENCH

Sauce Bourguignonne

1 C minced onion
1 C peeled and diced carrots
1/2 C diced celery (optional)
3 cloves garlic, pressed or minced
3 C water (or 2 C water and 1 C red wine)
1 T tomato paste
1 C red wine
2 T red wine vinegar (or other vinegar)
Salt to taste
1 T chopped fresh rosemary (or 1 t dried)
1/2 t dried thyme
1 t dried basil
1/2 t pepper
1/3 C cold water
2 T arrowroot powder (or cornstarch)

Sauté onion, carrots, celery, and garlic in 2 teaspoons water for
5 min. Place in a heavy 3 quart pot along with remaining
ingredients except 1/3 cup of water and arrowroot. Bring to a
boil, cover partially, and simmer for 15 – 20 min., until
vegetables are tender.

Whisk together cold water and arrowroot until smooth and
fully dissolved. Slowly pour into simmering sauce, stirring
constantly. Lower heat and continue stirring as sauce thickens
and becomes shiny, about 5 min. If necessary, add more
dissolved arrowroot, a teaspoon at a time, until sauce reaches
desired consistency. Serve over Chickpea-couscous . Also good
over rice, pasta, or potatoes.

Chickpea-Couscous Croquettes

2 C cooked and drained chickpeas (or equivalent canned)
1 C uncooked couscous
1/2 C tomato juice
1/2 C dry red wine
3 T soy sauce
2 T Dijon mustard
2 T red wine vinegar
2 t dried rosemary
1 t dried thyme
1/2 t black pepper
3 T minced fresh parsley
3 or more cloves garlic, pressed
1/2 – 1 T olive oil

Process chickpeas with a hand blender or food processor until relatively smooth.

In a heavy 1 quart pot, combine couscous, tomato juice, and red wine. Stir and bring to a boil. Lower heat, cover, and simmer for 3 min., until couscous has absorbed all liquid. Let sit for 5 min.

Add cooked couscous to chickpea mixture along with remaining ingredients except oil. Mix well.

Lightly oil your hands. Shape 2 – 3 tablespoons of mixture into about 24 balls. Flatten to form patties about 2 inches wide and 1/2 inch thick.

Brush patties with olive oil, if desired, and place on a lightly oiled baking tray. Bake for 15 min. at 350, turn over, brush with oil, and bake for another 10-12 min.

(Or, simply spread chickpea mixture in a lightly oiled baking pan and bake at 350° for 30 min. Cut into wedges, serve with Sauce Bourguignonne and a green salad.)

The Most Noble Diet

Ratatouille

4 garlic cloves, chopped
Oil or water for sautéing
1 med. eggplant in 1 inch cubes
3 zucchini, cubed
2 sliced green peppers
1 sliced onion
3 tomatoes, chunked
1 t oregano
1 bay leaf
salt and pepper to taste

Salt eggplant liberally and set aside for about 20 minutes. (Salt pulls the bitterness out.) Rinse thoroughly.

Sauté garlic, set aside. Sauté eggplant and zucchini, set aside. Sauté other vegetables and bay leaf, adding garlic and salt/pepper. Layer all in casserole dish, removing bay leaf. Bake 1 hour at 300°

Vegetables Provencal

2 small zucchini
1/2 lb. eggplant
1/2 lb. tomatoes (fresh or canned)
1 med. bell pepper, seeded
1 small red onion
1/4 lb. mushrooms (optional)
1/2 C water
1 clove garlic, minced
1 T tomato paste
1/4 C chopped fresh parsley
2 t basil
1 t minced fresh thyme or 1/2 t dried
1/2 t minced fresh rosemary or 1/4 t dried
freshly ground pepper to taste
balsamic vinegar (optional)

Cut all vegetables into 1/2 in. cubes. Place water in large, heavy pot. Add garlic and tomato paste. Heat and stir until well mixed. Add vegetables, cover, and cook until tender but not mushy, about 15 min. Stir in herbs and season with plenty of pepper. Serve warm and cold, splashing on some balsamic vinegar just before serving if desired. Serve over pasta or rice. Serves 4-6.

INDIAN

Baked Samosa Logs

5 cups diced cauliflower
1 1/3 cups fresh or frozen baby peas
1 1/2 T unsweetened coconut flakes
1 t curry powder
1/8 t cayenne (or 1/2 t paprika)
2 T chopped fresh cilantro
1 1/2 T lemon juice
1/2 t salt
12 whole wheat chapatis (or flour tortillas)
Olive oil spray or olive oil for brushing

Steam cauliflower in a large pan for 10 minutes. If using frozen peas, defrost; add peas and steam for 3 more minutes. Transfer cauliflower and peas to a bowl and add coconut, curry powder, cayenne or paprika, cilantro, lemon juice and salt. Toss to mix. Allow mixture to cool slightly.

Preheat oven to 375°. Place one chapati on a work surface and brush lightly with water. Place about 1/2 cup filling in the middle of the chapati. Fold ends over like an enchilada.. Place in a baking dish, seam side down. Repeat for remaining chapatis. (This is kind of messy.) Pour any remaining filling on top.

Bake for 15 to 20 minutes. Serve with Fruit-Sweetened Tomato Chutney or other chutney. Samosas can be made a day ahead of time and baked just before serving. They reheat well in the microwave. Serves 6.

Fruit-Sweetened Tomato Chutney

2 t olive oil (or water)
2 T freshly grated ginger root
1/2 T minced jalapeño pepper
1 t cumin seeds, crushed (or ground cumin)
1/2 T coriander seeds, crushed
1 1/2 cups tomato purée
2 cups diced tomatoes, with juice
1/2 cup white grape juice concentrate (undiluted)
Salt and freshly ground pepper to taste

Heat oil or water in a large saucepan. Add ginger, pepper, and cumin and coriander seeds. Cook until fragrant, about 1 – 2 minutes. Add remaining ingredients and bring mixture to a boil. Reduce heat and simmer, uncovered, for 35 – 40 min. About 1 1/2 cups.

Chutney can be made 1 or 2 days in advance; store in refrigerator. If doubling recipe, increase cooking time by 15 min. If freezing chutney, season with salt and pepper before serving.

Aloo Gajjar

2 T vegetable oil
1 t whole cumin seed (or ground cumin)
2 med. potatoes, diced
3 med. carrots, diced
1 t chili powder or cayenne pepper
1 t ground coriander
1/4 t ground turmeric
salt to taste
juice of half a lemon

Heat oil, add cumin seeds and cook until the start to pop, add potatoes. Cook 3 – 4 minutes, add carrots and spices. Cook another couple of minutes, sprinkling with water and cover. Cook for 10 min. until vegetables are done, sprinkle with lemon juice. Serves 2.

Indian Vegetable Stew

1 T safflower oil
2 cloves garlic, minced
1 1/2 T fresh minced ginger root
1 t ground cumin
1/2 t ground coriander
1/4 t ground cloves
1/2 t ground cardamom
1/4 t ground mustard
1/2 t ground turmeric
1/2 t cinnamon
1 t salt
3 C vegetable broth or water
3 T lime or lemon juice
1 T fructose or other sugar
3 carrots, peeled and sliced diagonally
2 C cauliflower florets
2 medium potatoes, diced

In a large saucepan, sauté garlic and ginger in oil for 1 min. Add cumin, coriander, cloves, cardamom, mustard, turmeric, cinnamon, and salt. Stir and cook for 2 min. to release flavors. Add broth, juice, and fructose and continue cooking for 3 – 4 min. Add vegetables and cook, covered, until tender, about 25 min. Serve with rice or bread. Makes 4 servings.

The Most Noble Diet

Curried Potatoes, Cauliflower, and Peas

2 t oil
2 medium baking potatoes, cut into 1/2 inch cubes
1 large onion, finely chopped
1 small cauliflower, cut into florets
1 large carrot, finely chopped
1 T curry powder
1/2 t ground cumin
1/2 t turmeric
Pinch of cayenne pepper
1 C vegetable stock, vegetable bouillon, or water
1 C fresh (or thawed frozen) peas
3 T soy sauce

Heat oil in large skillet over medium heat. Add potatoes, onion, and carrot, and cook, stirring often, until the potatoes are lightly browned, about 8 min.

Add the cauliflower, curry powder, cumin, turmeric, and cayenne and stir for 30 sec. Add stock, reduce heat and cover. Simmer 10 min., stirring occasionally.

Stir in peas and soy sauce, and cook, uncovered, until the liquid has thickened, about 2 min. Makes 4 servings

ITALIAN

Minestrone

2 C shell or other eggless macaroni
1 T olive oil
1 medium onion, chopped
1 medium carrot, chopped
1 medium rib celery, with leaves, chopped
4 garlic gloves, minced
8 C vegetable stock or vegetable bouillon
3 medium tomatoes, finely chopped, or 1 14 oz. can
unsweetened Italian tomatoes, undrained, chopped
1 medium potato, unpeeled, cut into 1/2 inch pieces
1 t dried rosemary
2 t dried basil
1 t dried oregano
1 bay leaf
1/2 t salt
1/4 t freshly ground black pepper
3 C finely shredded green cabbage (1/2 small head)
1/2 C finely chopped fresh parsley

In a medium pot of lightly salted boiling water, cook noodles until just tender, about 6 min. Drain, rinse under cold water, and drain again. Set the noodles aside.

In a large pot, heat the olive oil over medium heat. Add onion, carrot, celery, and garlic, and cook, stirring occasionally, until softened, about 5 min.

Stir in the vegetable stock, tomatoes, potato, rosemary, basil, oregano, bay leaf, salt, and pepper. Bring to a simmer and cook, partially covered, until the potatoes are almost tender, about 8 min.

Stir in cabbage and parsley and simmer, partially covered, until the cabbage is tender, about 15 min. Stir in cooked noodles and simmer until heated through, about 5 min. Remove bay leaf and serve immediately.

Stuffed Peppers

2 C water
1 C long-grain brown rice
8 large green bell peppers

Tomato Sauce:
1 T olive oil or water
1 small onion, finely chopped
2 garlic cloves, minced
16 oz can unsweetened tomatoes, undrained, coarsely chopped
6 oz can unsweetened tomato paste
1 t dried basil
1 t dried oregano
1/2 t dried thyme
1 t fine sea salt
1/4 t freshly ground black pepper

1 t olive oil or water
1 medium onion, chopped
1 C chopped mushrooms
1 med. zucchini, chopped
2 garlic cloves, minced

In a medium saucepan, bring water to boil over high heat. Add rice, cover, reduce heat and simmer until the water is absorbed, 30 – 40 min. Transfer rice to a large bowl.

Put one inch of water into a large saucepan with a steamer basket, cover with the lid, and bring to a boil. Carefully trim the bottoms of the peppers so they sit straight. Slice off the tops and carefully remove the seeds and ribs with your fingers. (Save the tops for chopping and using in another recipe.) Put the peppers in the steamer basket, cover, and steam peppers until they are bright green but still firm, 5 – 8 min. Remove from the steamer and set aside.

Preheat oven to 350°. Lightly oil a 9 x 13 inch baking dish. In a medium saucepan, heat the oil or water over medium heat. Add onion and garlic and cook, stirring often, until softened, about 5 min. Stir in the tomatoes with juice, tomato paste, basil, oregano, thyme, salt, and pepper.   Bring to a simmer, reduce the heat to low, and cook until slightly thickened, about 20 min. Remove from heat.

Meanwhile, heat olive oil or water in large frying pan over medium heat. Add onion, mushrooms, zucchini, and garlic and cook until the mushrooms are lightly browned, about 8 min. Add to the rice.

Add 1/2 cup of tomato sauce to the rice and vegetables and mix well. Fill the bell pepper cups with the tomato-rice mixture. Put the stuffed peppers into the prepared baking dish. Pour the remaining tomato sauce on and around the peppers. Bake until bubbling, 20 – 30 min. Serve immediately. Serves 8.

Red Sauce

1 small onion, minced
3 large cloves garlic, minced
1/3 C dry red wine
3 1/2 C tomato puree (28 oz can)
1 1/2 C canned whole peeled tomatoes, coarsely chopped, with juice
1 whole carrot, peeled
1 green pepper, chopped
1 T minced fresh parsley
1 T dried basil
1 bay leaf
2 t dried oregano
1/4 t dried rosemary
1/8 t salt

Briefly sauté onions, and garlic in a little of the wine, then add remaining wine, and the green pepper, cover, and simmer for 10 min. If more liquid is needed, use the juice from the canned tomatoes. Add remaining ingredients and continue simmering, uncovered, 30 – 45 minutes longer, or until sauce is thick and flavors have melded. If time permits, let the sauce sit overnight in the refrigerator. Before serving, discard bay leaf and carrot. Serve over pasta. (or rice, or potatoes)

Lasagna

1 lb. lasagna noodles

Tofu Ricotta:
1 lb. firm tofu
2 T olive oil
salt
1/2 t nutmeg

Filling:
5 cloves garlic
2 large zucchini, sliced thinly (approx. 4 c)
2 t basil
2 t oregano
1 t paprika
salt and pepper
2 10 oz. boxes frozen chopped spinach (or equivalent fresh, wilted, chopped)

1-2 cans (27 oz each) spaghetti sauce, depending on how much sauce you like.

Prepare lasagna noodles. Rinse under cold water and lay out on paper towels or waxed paper. Cover with a towel to prevent drying.

Prepare ricotta by combining ingredients with a food processor or hand blender.

Sauté zucchini and garlic in several T water with spices.

Steam spinach until defrosted. Squeeze out excess water.

Preheat oven to 350°. Brush a 9x13 baking dish with olive oil. Pour a thin layer of spaghetti sauce on bottom, layer a row of noodles, ricotta, and then veggies and more seasonings. Repeat twice, ending with noodles, ricotta, and spaghetti sauce. Sprinkle with basil, oregano, and paprika. Bake 45 minutes.

Pasta Primavera

Vegetable mixture
1 T olive oil
1 onion chopped
2 cloves garlic, minced
1/2 lb. mushrooms, washed and sliced
1 t oregano
1 t basil
1/2 t thyme
1 bell pepper, diced
1/4 C fresh chopped parsley
2 med. zucchini, diced
4 large tomatoes, finely chopped
1/2 t salt

Sauce
2 T margarine
2 T flour
1 C soymilk

1 lb. eggless fettucini or other pasta

1/4 C finely chopped toasted almonds (optional)

Sauté onion in olive oil for 2 min., then add the garlic,
mushrooms, and herbs. Cook until mushrooms are brown.
Add bell pepper, parsley, zucchini, and tomatoes and cook until
pepper is tender/crisp, 3 – 5 min. Add salt to taste.

In a separate pan, melt the margarine and stir in the flour.
Cook 30 sec. Whisk in soymilk and cook over medium heat,
stirring constantly until thickened.

Cook pasta according to package instructions, until just
tender. Place in baking dish, and sprinkle with salt and pepper.
Spread while sauce over pasta, then top with vegetable
mixture. Sprinkle with toasted almonds if desired. Bake at 350°
for 20 min.

The Most Noble Diet

Vegetable Stifado

1 t olive oil
2 cloves garlic, sliced
2 onions, chopped
2 med. potatoes, thinly sliced
1 t ground cinnamon
1 t cumin seeds
1/4 t cayenne pepper
juice of 1 lemon
2 carrots, cut into sticks
12-16 oz can crushed tomatoes
1 can kidney beans (1 1/2 C cooked beans)
1 head broccoli, broken into flowerets
salt and pepper to taste

In a heavy-bottomed pan, sauté onions and garlic in oil or water. Add potatoes, spices, and lemon juice, cover and cook 5 min. Add carrots and tomatoes, cook 30 min., stirring occasionally. Add beans, broccoli, salt and pepper, and cook 10 min. Serve with rice and a green salad.

MISCELLANEOUS

Quick Breads

Simple variety "breads" cam be made by mixing whole grain flour (about 2 T for each slice desired) with luke warm water and a pinch of yeast. Let sit for about 15 minutes then add one or more of the following: nutritional years, spices, herbs, grated vegetables, dried fruits. Place on a non-stick cookie sheet in large cookie size portions. Bake about 25 minutes at 325°. Remove carefully with wooden spatula. This can also be used for pizza crust. (see below)

The Most Noble Pizza

Use Quick breads recipe, adjusting amount for size of pizza you wish to make. Spread dough with floured hand onto floured baking sheet. Bake at 325 ° for 8 minutes then top with sauce and toppings (such as bell peppers, onions, garlic, broccoli, spinach, mushrooms, nutritional yeast) . Bake 10 more min..

Gourmet Garlic Bread

Most garlic bread is high in fat because butter or margarine is used as a vehicle to spread the garlic. Garlic itself will spread easily if baked. Bake whole cloves of unpeeled garlic at 325° for 20 min. until easily pierced with a fork. The inside should be a creamy consistency. Spread on bread and toast or broil for 2 1/2 minutes.

Spicy Bulghar Pilaf

2 T oil
1 med. onion, chopped
2 cloves garlic, minced
1 C bulghar wheat
2 t chili powder
3/4 t ground cumin
1/2 red (or other) bell pepper, finely diced
1/2 t salt
1 1/2 C boiling vegetable stock or water

Sauté onion, garlic, and bulghar for 2 – 3 min. Stir in chili powder and cumin, and continue cooking for 2 min.

Add bell pepper and salt, then pour in the boiling stock or water. Bring to a boil, then reduce to a simmer. Cover and cook, without stirring, until all liquid is absorbed (about 20 min.). Good with Mexican dishes, in place of rice.

Falafel

1 C dried chick peas, soaked overnight in 4 C water
1 t baking soda
1 t salt
1 medium onion
1 t ground cumin
1 t ground coriander
2 cloves garlic
1 T lemon juice
2 T parsley
dash cayenne pepper

Drain the chickpeas and process them lightly in a food processor or blender. Add remaining ingredients and process further until the mixture is the texture of coarse breadcrumbs. Form patties and "fry" in a little oil in a frying pan. For a lower-fat version, try baking the patties on a lightly oiled baking sheet at 350 for 20 min. Serve with hummus (your favorite) in pita bread, with sliced cucumbers and tomatoes.

Bean Spread ("Refried" Beans)

1 lb. pinto or black beans (dried)
1 head garlic, chopped (more or less to taste)
1 T cumin
1/2 C salsa
2 T lemon juice

Other spices to taste: oregano, basil, parsley, pepper, salt.

Place beans in large pot, cover with water. Soak overnight, at least 6 hours. Drain, cover with fresh water. Bring to a boil and then simmer until very tender (1 hour) Drain. Blend with a hand mixer or blender until very smooth. Add remaining ingredients, blend again until very smooth. Allow flavors to absorb in refrigerator. Use as a sandwich spread or bean dip, or reheat and use as a filling for tacos, burritos, and other Mexican dishes.

Shepherd's Pie

4 large potatoes, sliced
1/2 C soymilk
1/2 t salt

1 T olive oil
2 onions, chopped
1 large bell pepper, diced
2 carrots, sliced
2 stalks of celery, sliced
2 C cauliflower (or mushrooms)
1 can chopped tomatoes (or 4 large tomatoes, diced)
2 C cooked kidney (or chili) beans (15 oz can), drained
1/2 t paprika
1/2 t black pepper
2 T soy sauce

Dice potatoes, then steam over boiling water until tender. Mash with soymilk and salt. Set aside.

In a large skillet, sauté onions, pepper, carrot, and celery for 3 min. over medium heat. Add cauliflower or mushrooms, cover pan and cook for an additional 7 min., stirring occasionally. Add tomatoes, kidney beans, paprika, and soy sauce, then cover and cook 10 – 15 min.

Put vegetables into a 9 x 13 inch baking dish and spread mashed potatoes evenly over the top. Sprinkle with paprika. Bake at 350° for 25 min., until hot and bubbly. Serves 8.

DESSERTS

Apple Cake

1/2 C raisins
1 apple, chopped
1 C water
1/2 C turbinado sugar
1/2 t salt
2 t cinnamon
1 t ginger
3/4 t nutmeg
1/4 t cloves
2 C whole wheat pastry flour
    (or 1 1/2 C flour + 1 C Nutrigrain or bran cereal)
1 t baking powder
1 t baking soda

Combine fruits, sugar, water and seasonings in a large saucepan and bring to a boil. Continue boiling for 2 min. , stirring, then remove from heat and cool completely.

    When fruit mixture is cool, mix in dry ingredients. Spread into a round cake pan (greased and floured, if not non-stick) and bake at 350° for 40 min. or until a toothpick inserted into the center comes out clean.

Blueberry Crisp

2 C cooked rice or bulghur
3/4 C soymilk
1/4 C fructose or other sugar
1 t cinnamon
3 C fresh or frozen blueberries

Preheat oven to 350°. In a bowl, combine rice or bulghur, soymilk, sugar, and cinnamon. Add fruit and mix gently. Transfer to an 8 in. square baking pan and cover with foil. Bake 30 min., cool slightly before serving.

Carob Cake

2 1/3 C whole-wheat flour
1 C water
1/2 C soymilk
1 T egg replacer
2/3 C carob powder
1 T grain "coffee"
1 C Fruitsource, or 1 C maple syrup
1 t vanilla
2 1/2 t baking powder

Preheat oven to 350°. Mix 1/3 C flour with 1 C water. Cook in a small saucepan until thick. Cool.

Mix soymilk, egg replacer, carob powder and grain coffee with wire whisk or mixer. Beat together sweetener, flour and water mixture, and vanilla in another bowl. Add to carob mixture. Combine remaining 2 C flour and baking powder. Add to above ingredients.

Bake in a 9 or 10-inch square oiled pan for 35-40 minutes, or until knife inserted comes out clean. (This cake is not low calorie.)

Can be frosted with the following, but with the frosting, it is no longer low fat:
8-10 oz. medium tofu
2 T grain "coffee"
5 T carob powder
1/4 C maple syrup and 1/4 C fructose
(OR 1/2 C maple syrup OR 1/2 C Fruitsource)

Blend in a blender or with a hand mixture until smooth. This may take a while. Spread on cake when still slightly warm (but not hot) because this frosting tends to thicken up. (Refrigerate remaining cake, if there is any.)

The Most Noble Diet

Pumpkin Spice Cake

1 1/4 C unbleached white flour or whole-wheat pastry flour
1 1/2 t ground cinnamon
1/2 t ground nutmeg
1 t pumpkin pie spice (cloves, allspice)
1 t baking powder
1/2 t baking soda
1/2 t salt
1 C Grape Nuts, Nutrigrain, or bran cereal
3/4 C soymilk
1 T egg replacer
2/3 C turbinado or other sugar
3/4 C pumpkin purée
1/4 C raisins

Preheat oven to 400°. Lightly oil a cake pan and dust with flower. Shake out excess flower.

In a large bowl, combine flour, cinnamon, nutmeg, pumpkin pie spice, baking powder, baking soda, sugar, and salt. Add cereal, and toss to coat. In another bowl, whisk together soymilk, Egg Replacer, and pumpkin purée. Stir in raisins.

Combine contents of both bowls, folding until just incorporated. Spoon batter into 9x9 pan or loaf pan. Bake for 25 min., then lower heat to 300° and bake for 10 min. more, or until a toothpick inserted into the center comes out clean.

Carrot Cake

1 C unsweetened applesauce
1 C turbinado or other sugar
1 1/2 C soymilk
2 C unbleached white and 2 C whole wheat flour
2 t baking powder
2 t baking soda
1 t salt
2 t cinnamon
1 t allspice
3 C grated carrots
1/2 C raisins

Preheat oven to 350°. Combine applesauce, sugar, and soymilk in large bowl. In another bowl, combine flours, baking powder, baking soda, salt, cinnamon, and allspice, add to applesauce mixture. Stir in carrots and raisins.

Grease and flour 2 cake pans (or use non-stick) and pour in batter. Bake for 50 min., until toothpick inserted into center comes out clean. "Frost" with applebutter, if desired.

Sweet Potato (or Pumpkin) Pie

2 C sweet potato (or pumpkin)
1 C soymilk
3/4 C turbinado or other sugar
1 T molasses
1/2 t salt
1/2 t nutmeg
1/2 t ginger
1/2 t cloves
1 t cornstarch

Combine all with blender or mixer. Pour into unbaked pie crust. Bake for 10 min. at 425°, reduce heat to 350° and bake for 40-50 min. longer. Good for the winter holidays.

Notes

Notes

Notes